CANCER IN ELDERLY PEOPLE

WORKSHOP PROCEEDINGS

National Cancer Policy Forum

INSTITUTE OF MEDICINE
OF THE NATIONAL ACADEMIES

THE NATIONAL ACADEMIES PRESS
Washington, D.C.
www.nap.edu

THE NATIONAL ACADEMIES PRESS   500 Fifth Street, N.W.   Washington, DC 20001

NOTICE: The project that is the subject of this report was approved by the Governing Board of the National Research Council, whose members are drawn from the councils of the National Academy of Sciences, the National Academy of Engineering, and the Institute of Medicine.

This study was supported by Contracts No. HHSN261200611002C, 200-2005-13434, TO #1, HHSM-500-2005-00179P, HHSP23320042509XI, TO #4, 223-01-2460, TO #27, HHSH25056133, TO #6 between the National Academy of Sciences and, respectively, the National Cancer Institute, the Centers for Disease Control and Prevention, the Centers for Medicare and Medicaid Services, the Agency for Healthcare Research and Quality, the Food and Drug Administration, and the Health Resources and Services Administration. Support was also received from the American Cancer Society, the American Society of Clinical Oncology, and C-Change. Any opinions, findings, conclusions, or recommendations expressed in this publication are those of the author(s) and do not necessarily reflect the view of the organizations or agencies that provided support for this project.

International Standard Book Number-13: 978-0-309-10476-0
International Standard Book Number-10: 0-309-10476-9

Additional copies of this report are available from the National Academies Press, 500 Fifth Street, N.W., Lockbox 285, Washington, DC 20055; (800) 624-6242 or (202) 334-3313 (in the Washington metropolitan area); Internet, **http://www.nap.edu.**

For more information about the Institute of Medicine, visit the IOM home page at: **www.iom.edu**

Printed in the United States of America.

The serpent has been a symbol of long life, healing, and knowledge among almost all cultures and religions since the beginning of recorded history. The serpent adopted as a logotype by the Institute of Medicine is a relief carving from ancient Greece, now held by the Staatliche Museen in Berlin.

Suggested citation: Institute of Medicine (IOM). 2007. *Cancer in elderly people: Workshop proceedings.* Washington, DC: The National Academies Press.

"Knowing is not enough; we must apply. Willing is not enough; we must do."

—Goethe

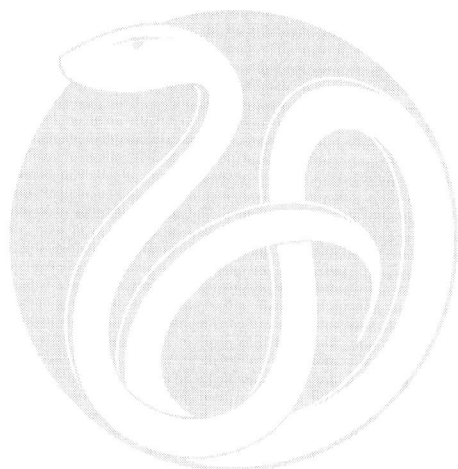

INSTITUTE OF MEDICINE
OF THE NATIONAL ACADEMIES

Advising the Nation. Improving Health.

THE NATIONAL ACADEMIES
Advisers to the Nation on Science, Engineering, and Medicine

The **National Academy of Sciences** is a private, nonprofit, self-perpetuating society of distinguished scholars engaged in scientific and engineering research, dedicated to the furtherance of science and technology and to their use for the general welfare. Upon the authority of the charter granted to it by the Congress in 1863, the Academy has a mandate that requires it to advise the federal government on scientific and technical matters. Dr. Ralph J. Cicerone is president of the National Academy of Sciences.

The **National Academy of Engineering** was established in 1964, under the charter of the National Academy of Sciences, as a parallel organization of outstanding engineers. It is autonomous in its administration and in the selection of its members, sharing with the National Academy of Sciences the responsibility for advising the federal government. The National Academy of Engineering also sponsors engineering programs aimed at meeting national needs, encourages education and research, and recognizes the superior achievements of engineers. Dr. Wm. A. Wulf is president of the National Academy of Engineering.

The **Institute of Medicine** was established in 1970 by the National Academy of Sciences to secure the services of eminent members of appropriate professions in the examination of policy matters pertaining to the health of the public. The Institute acts under the responsibility given to the National Academy of Sciences by its congressional charter to be an adviser to the federal government and, upon its own initiative, to identify issues of medical care, research, and education. Dr. Harvey V. Fineberg is president of the Institute of Medicine.

The **National Research Council** was organized by the National Academy of Sciences in 1916 to associate the broad community of science and technology with the Academy's purposes of furthering knowledge and advising the federal government. Functioning in accordance with general policies determined by the Academy, the Council has become the principal operating agency of both the National Academy of Sciences and the National Academy of Engineering in providing services to the government, the public, and the scientific and engineering communities. The Council is administered jointly by both Academies and the Institute of Medicine. Dr. Ralph J. Cicerone and Dr. Wm. A. Wulf are chair and vice chair, respectively, of the National Research Council.

www.national-academies.org

NATIONAL CANCER POLICY FORUM

JANET WOODCOCK, Deputy Commissioner for Operations, Food and Drug Administration

Staff

SHARYL NASS, Senior Program Officer
ROGER HERDMAN, Director, National Cancer Policy Forum
ALIZA NORWOOD, Research Assistant
MARY ANN PRYOR, Senior Program Assistant

This volume has been reviewed in draft form in accordance with procedures approved by the NRC's Report Review Committee. We wish to thank Betty Ferrell, Ph.D., FAAN, for her review and Clyde Behney for serving as coordinator of the review.

Contents

1   Introduction   1

2   Prepared Presentations and Discussion   3

References   92

Appendix: Workshop Agenda   97

1

Introduction

Proceedings of a workshop presented to the Institute of Medicine's (IOM) National Cancer Policy Forum (NCPF) on October 30, 2006, are the result of discussions at a previous meeting on June 16, 2006. That discussion, led by NCPF members Betty Ferrell and Patricia Ganz, noted that a high proportion of cancer occurs primarily in older persons. Incidence of the major cancers increases with advancing age. Moreover, the expansion of the aging population of the United States will likely have far-reaching effects on the health status of Americans and the nation's health-care system, particularly in persons 65 and older. Drs. Ferrell and Ganz proposed that the NCPF could provide a useful review of the various important implications of changing demographics and the cancer disease burden in the United States. They volunteered to work with staff to organize and lead a workshop on the subject. The agenda is reproduced in the appendix to these proceedings. Chapter 2 includes presentations of scheduled speakers as well as comments from speakers, NCPF members, and invited participants. The transcriptions are edited to eliminate redundancy and grammatical errors. Selections from PowerPoint presentations are added to the text to clarify speakers' messages.

This workshop was a major part of the regularly scheduled meeting of the NCPF. The NCPF was established as a unit of the IOM on May 1, 2005, with support from the National Cancer Institute, the Centers for Disease Control and Prevention, the Agency for Healthcare Research and Quality, the Food and Drug Administration, the Centers for Medicare and

Medicaid Services, the Health Resources and Services Administration, the American Cancer Society, the American Society of Clinical Oncology, C-Change, and UnitedHealth Group. The NCPF is a successor to the National Cancer Policy Board (1997–2005); it is designed to provide 22 governmental, industry, academic, and other members a venue for exchanging information and presenting individual views on emerging policy issues in the nation's effort to combat cancer. Publication of these proceedings not only informs the NCPF, it also provides an opportunity to make the information and views presented and discussed available to a broad public audience. Deliberations actually communicated within the workshop are reported without additional comment, interpretation, or analysis. These proceedings may serve as an opening to additional IOM study in the future.

2

Prepared Presentations and Discussion

Dr. Patricia Ganz, Professor of Medicine, University of California, Los Angeles: Just over 20 years ago the National Cancer Institute (NCI) issued its first request for application (RFA): Patterns of Care for Elderly Cancer Patients: Implications for Cancer Control, 1983. This RFA was a direct result of the work of our first invited speaker, Rosemary Yancik, who was then at the NCI. Research conducted as part of that RFA demonstrated that older patients received poorer quality of care, even when they did not have comorbid conditions. Furthermore, studies through the NCI's Cooperative Trials Groups documented consistent underrepresentation of elderly people in clinical trials. Indeed, standards of eligibility specifically excluded people over 65 years of age. Eventually, as discrimination against elderly people became an issue in general, these problems began to be recognized. The Medicare Hospice Benefit did not exist at that time. Rehabilitation primarily involved helping the recovery of patients who had radical surgery (e.g., radical mastectomy, amputation, or laryngectomy). The focus was on inpatient hospitalizations, which in that era were quite prolonged.

Where are we today? Unfortunately, older cancer patients still do not receive standard care, in spite of nearly universal health insurance for that population through Medicare. Older cancer patients continue to be underrepresented in clinical trials. Hospice care is covered by the Centers for Medicare and Medicaid Services (CMS), but referral often occurs very late in the course of illness, possibly because of patient or physician reluctance. In contrast to 20 years ago, most cancer care today occurs in the outpatient setting. There has been a dearth of interest in cancer rehabilitation services mostly because reimbursement for outpatients has not been supported. Thus, because of the outpatient locus and complexity of care, there is a high burden on families, particularly if one is a member of the "sandwich generation" (i.e., a person taking care of a parent).

Despite this state of affairs, data show there have been gradual improvements in survival of older people with cancer, although these improvements lag far behind those made in pediatric oncology. Sixty percent of survivors are currently over age 65. Even if they were not diagnosed when they were older, they are living into their older years. Breast, prostate, and colon cancers are the three most prevalent cancer sites. Approximately 14 percent of the 10.5 million estimated cancer survivors were diagnosed over 20 years ago. They are often living with complications of treatments that at the time were much more radical and much more toxic than procedures of today.

Some final thoughts as we begin our discussion: I think the older cancer patient provides an opportunity for us to think of all the issues that we face in cancer care, including quality of care, access to care, survivorship concerns, and end of life. I am grateful to the leadership and members of the NCPF for encouraging discussion on this topic. I think the speakers today will give us a glimpse of all of these issues in a very important context—our older cancer patient population.

Dr. Betty Ferrell, Research Scientist, City of Hope National Medical Center: In the National Cancer Policy Forum (NCPF), we tend to think inclusively about whatever topic we discuss: What are the quality-of-care issues? What are the issues of access, of diversity, and the underserved? What are the problems across the trajectory from diagnoses through end-of-life care? And what is the financial burden on our health-care system and on the individual? I do not think there is any other topic that could be tackled that could cross all of those areas as well as cancer in elderly people.

In addition, so often we select a topic and deal with it because it is a current crisis, but addressing cancer in elderly people gives us an opportunity, as Dr. Ganz has shown, to be thinking ahead. If we project 5 or 10 years from now, clearly the demand on our system will be overwhelming. I think we have an opportunity, whatever the outcome of this workshop, to speak to the future and what challenges we will be facing.

Dr. Rosemary Yancik, Health Scientist Administrator, Geriatrics Branch, Geriatrics and Clinical Gerontology Program, National Institute on Aging, National Institutes of Health: The U.S. Demographic Imperative: Implications for Oncology Practice: Why an emphasis on cancer in the older person? According to the NCI Surveillance, Epidemiology, and End Results (SEER) Program data, persons aged 65 and older are at higher risk for most major malignancies. Coupled with this vulnerability, persons in this age group are also likely to have concomitant health problems also associated with advancing age (i.e., comorbidity). In Table 2-1, showing median ages of patients at diagnosis for both sexes, we observe that with the exception of non-Hodgkin's lymphoma (NHL), the median age in males for these common cancer sites is uniformly above the age of 65, and in some cases the median age is above 70 years. For females the situation is about the same for the tumors common to both men and women, and the total numbers for each sex are similar.

In Figure 2-1, the proportion of cancers in all sites in the 65 and older population is 56 percent; for many individual tumors, the proportions rise much higher.

TABLE 2-1 Median Age of Cancer Patients at Diagnosis, 2000–2003

Cancer Site	Male		Female	
	Median Age	Number	Median Age	Number
Breast	67	1,720	61	212,920
Colon	71	49,220	75	57,460
Corpus uteri	—	—	63	41,200
Leukemia	66	20,000	68	15,070
Lung	70	92,700	71	81,770
NHL*	64	30,680	69	28,190
Ovary	—	—	63	20,180
Pancreas	70	17,150	74	16,580
Prostate	68	230,110	—	—
Rectum	66	23,580	70	18,350
Stomach	70	13,400	74	8,880
Bladder	72	44,690	74	16,730
Total		523,350		517,330

*NHL = non-Hodgkin's lymphoma.

SOURCE: Adapted by Yancik from ACS Facts and Figures, 2006; NCI SEER Program Data, 2000–2003.

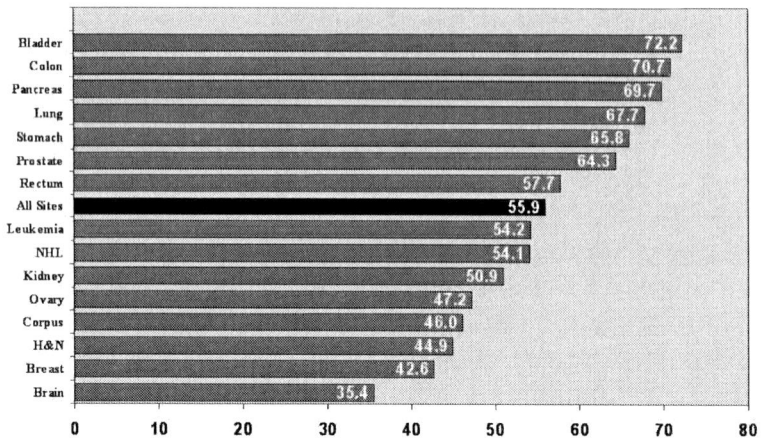

FIGURE 2-1 Proportion of tumors in patients 65 and older.
NOTE: Values reflect all races and both sexes.
NHL = non-Hodgkin's lymphoma.
SOURCE: Adapted by Yancik from NCI SEER Program Data, 2000–2003.

Figure 2-2 shows age-adjusted incidence and death rates for all cancer sites combined. The age-adjusted rate per 100,000 population, 2183.2, is 10 times greater for individuals 65 years and older as compared to 223.7, the rate for younger persons. Figure 2-3 shows the incidence for all sites in males and females. Age adjusted-death rates are 17 times greater for this age comparison with a rate of 64.2 for those ages less than 65 and 1096.4 for those age 65 and older. Figure 2-4 shows the latest SEER data for distribution of deaths at different ages for all-site cancers.

Age-specific differences from the NCI SEER Program for selected age groups further reveal distinctions along the aging continuum for males and females, all sites combined.

Figure 2-4 illustrates death rates throughout the age-group spectrum and displays the preponderance of the proportion of cancer deaths in the 65 and over population with a further delineation of that population into 65–74, 75–84, and 85 and over.

Figures 2-5 and 2-6, constructed from the same data sources for a subset of age groups, display the numbers of deaths for males and females caused by the four top common cancers—lung, colorectal, and either pros-

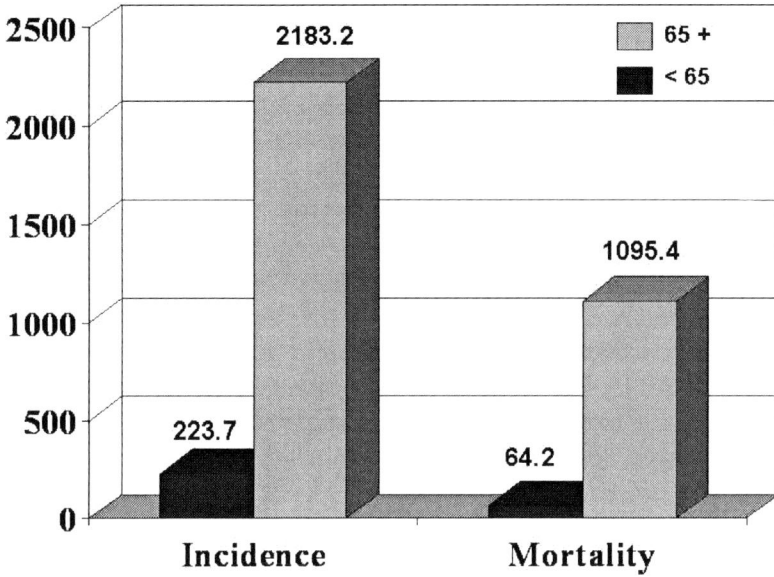

FIGURE 2-2 Age-adjusted incidence and death rates, all cancers.
SOURCE: Adapted by Yancik from NCI SEER Program Data 2000–2003.

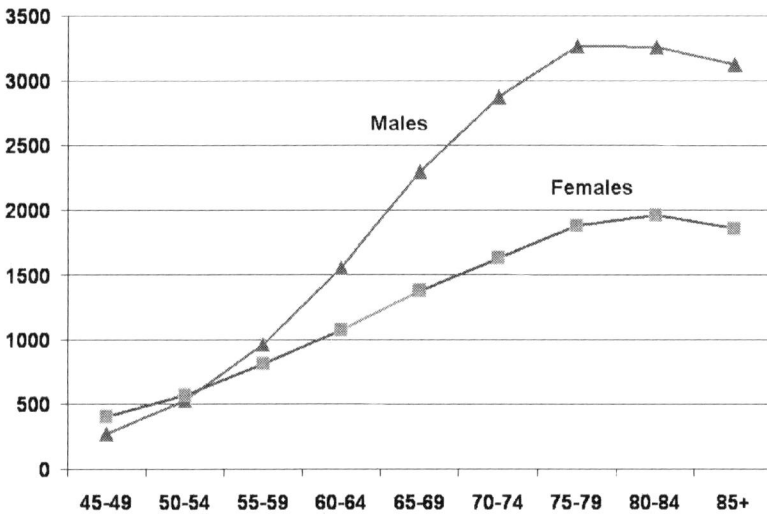

FIGURE 2-3 All-site cancer incidence rates by age and sex, 2000-2003.
SOURCE: Adapted by Yancik from NCI SEER Program Data 2000–2003.

N=564,830

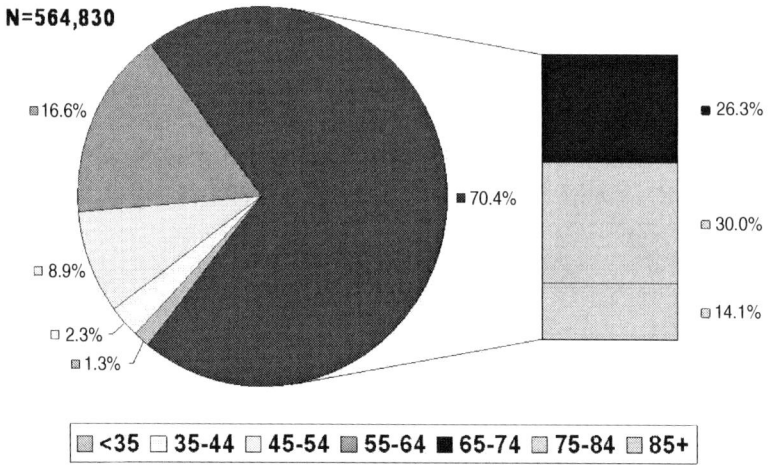

■ <35 ☐ 35-44 ☐ 45-54 ▨ 55-64 ■ 65-74 ▨ 75-84 ▨ 85+

FIGURE 2-4 Age distribution (%) of all-site cancer deaths, 2006.
SOURCE: Adapted by Yancik from the National Center for Health Statistics Death Estimates, U.S. Mortality Public Use Tapes, 1975–2003 as analyzed by the NCI SEER Program.

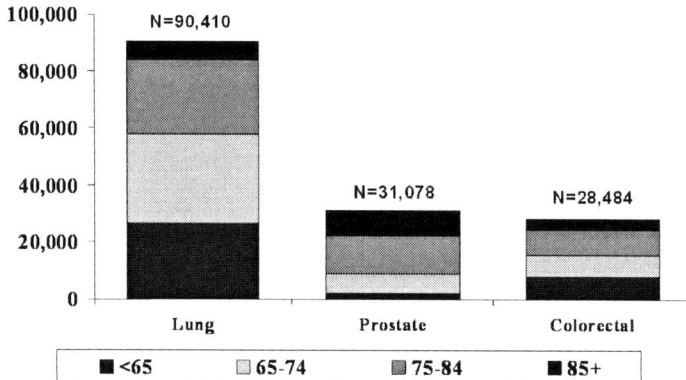

■ <65   ☐ 65-74   ▨ 75-84   ■ 85+

FIGURE 2-5 Male deaths for lung, prostate, and colorectal cancer by age, 2000.
SOURCE: Adapted by Yancik from NCI SEER Program Data, 2000–2003.

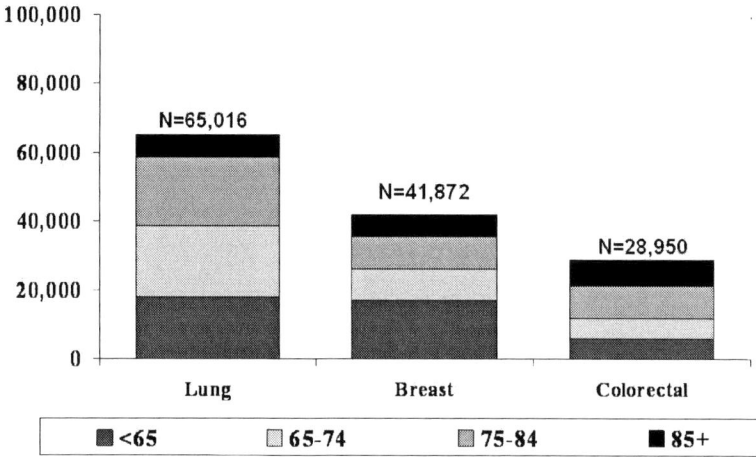

FIGURE 2-6 Female deaths for lung, breast, and colorectal cancer by age, 2000.
SOURCE: Adapted by Yancik from NCI SEER Program Data, 2000–2003.

tate or breast. The pattern of cancer prominence in older age groups is sustained with these data.

Who are the elderly, and what does "old" mean? Table 2-2 displays the life expectancies of Americans throughout the 1900s. In 1900, life expectancy was 46 years, with 11.5 years remaining for men at that age, and, for women, 48 with 12.2 years remaining. Progressing through the decades of the 20th century to the present, U.S. life expectancy is almost twice as high as it was in 1900. This is very important. We are aging within the aged in this country. There are more older persons than ever before in history. More older persons are surviving to the oldest ages, and by 2030 one in five, or 70 million, Americans will be 65 years or older.

Figure 2-7 displays how the population age pyramid of 1982 has gradually shifted to an age rectangle because of the aging of the 76 million baby boomers born between 1946 and 1964. In this context, the magnitude of the cancer burden in elderly people clearly requires our urgent attention. The Census Bureau projects the number of older people (those 65 or over) in the United States to reach over 70 million in 2030 with the oldest-old (age 85 years or older) projected to double by 2030 from 4.7 million to 9.6 million.

TABLE 2-2 U.S. Life Expectancy at Birth, 1900–2000 (Years Remaining)

Year	Men	Women
2000	74.1 (16.3)	79.5 (19.2)
1980	70.0	77.4
1960	66.6	73.1
1940	60.8	65.2
1920	53.6	54.6
1900	46.3 (11.5)	48.3 (12.2)

SOURCE: Adapted by Yancik from NCHS/U.S. Census Bureau, 2005.

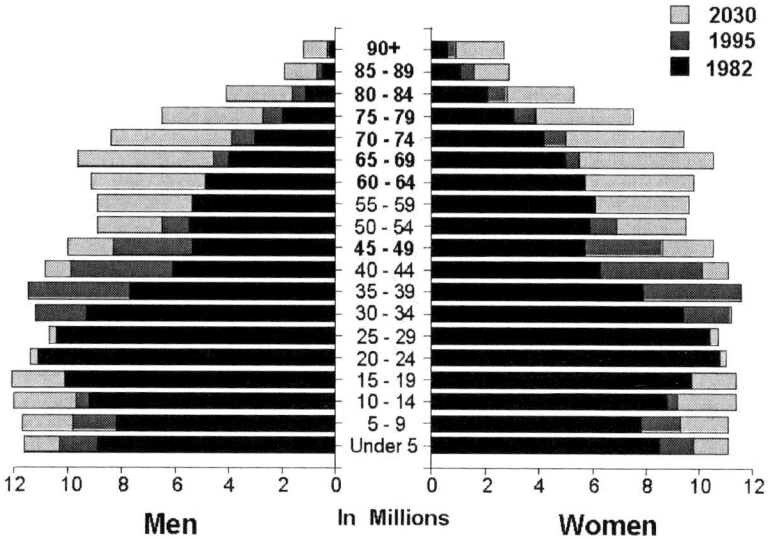

FIGURE 2-7 Expanding U.S. aging population.
SOURCE Adapted by Yancik from U.S. Census Bureau Current Population Reports P2-1104, 1993.

People are aging to older ages because in general they are healthier. The presence of comorbidities and cancer in older patients was mentioned earlier. The remainder of this presentation features data on female breast cancer which, after lung cancer, is the second highest cause of U.S. cancer deaths in women. According to most recent American Cancer Society data, about 41,000 deaths from breast cancer occurred in 2006.

In a National Institute on Aging (NIA)/NCI cancer and comorbidity collaborative study on the comorbidity burden of 1,800 breast cancer patients (using a population-based random sample of patients aged 55 to 101 years), my colleagues and I found that the number of comorbidities ranged from 0 to 13 per patient; the numbers of health problems increased with age (Yancik et al., 2001). With aging, physiological decrements and susceptibility to geriatric syndromes (incontinence and falls, among others) increase, as do chronic disease, susceptibility to infections, and other comorbidities. All of the major diseases and conditions common to older persons (e.g., heart-related conditions, diabetes, hypertension, chronic obstructive pulmonary diseases [COPD], cerebrovascular diseases, urinary tract problem, and subcategories of each were included in the study). Data were collected on the comorbidities of breast cancer patients by retrospective hospital record review. We also categorized by severity. The number of comorbidities for individual patients ranged from 0 to 13. Percentages are shown in Table 2-3: 263 patients (15 percent) died at or before the 30-month follow-up: from breast cancer (51.3 percent), heart disease (17 percent), or previous cancers (8.4 percent).

To briefly describe this sample of new breast cancer patients, 73 percent were diagnosed with stage I or II disease, 10 percent with stage III or

TABLE 2-3 Cause of Death in Breast Cancer Sample

	55–64	65–74	75–84	85+	Total
Breast cancer	48 (75.0)	33 (58.9)	38 (44.7)	16 (27.6)	135 (51.3)
Other cancers	4 (6.2)	6 (10.7)	9 (10.6)	3 (5.2)	22 (8.4)
Heart disease	4 (6.2)	4 (7.1)	18 (21.2)	19 (32.8)	45 (17.1)
Cerebrovascular	0	1 (1.8)	4 (13.8)	8 (13.8)	13 (4.0)
Digestive	1 (1.6)	1 (1.8)	3 (3.5)	4 (6.9)	9 (3.4)
Alzheimer/dementia	1 (1.6)	0	4 (4.7)	2 (3.4)	7 (2.7)
Pneumonia	0	0	2 (2.4)	3 (5.2)	5 (1.9)
COPD*/respiratory	1 (1.6)	2 (3.6)	1 (1.2)	1 (1.7)	13 (4.9)
Other	5 (7.8)	4 (7.1)	2 (2.4)	2 (3.4)	13 (4.9)
Unknown	0	5 (8.9)	4 (4.7)	0	9 (3.4)
Total deaths	64	56	85	58	263
Total patients	622	624	427	127	1800

*COPD = chronic obstructive pulmonary disease.
SOURCE: Adapted from Yancik et al., 2001.

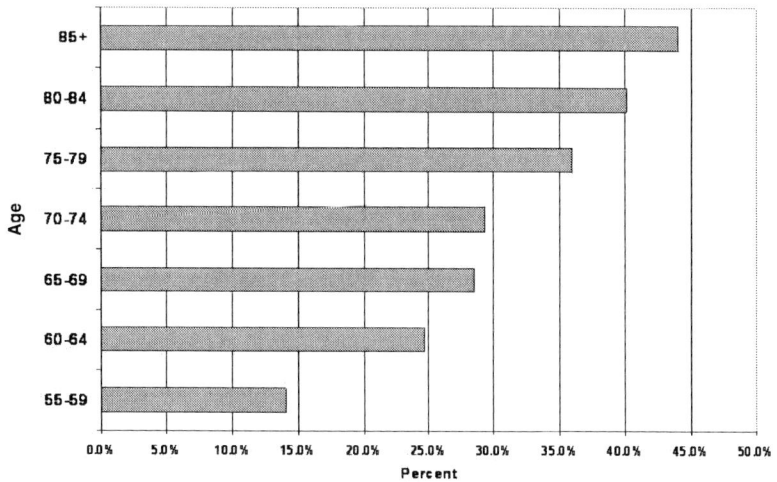

FIGURE 2-8 Frequency of breast cancer patients with one or more severe comorbidities by age.
SOURCE: Yancik et al., 2001.

IV, and 17 percent were not staged. Patients with stage I and II disease almost always (95 percent) received standard treatment, but patients in older age groups were less likely to receive therapy consistent with the National Institutes of Health (NIH) consensus statement or to have axillary dissections (and staging). Comorbidity, which increases in frequency in older patients, as shown in Figure 2-8, limits the ability to obtain prognostic information, tends to minimize treatment options, and increases the risk of death from causes other than breast cancer as shown for this NIA/ NCI study sample in Table 2-3, which summarizes the cause of death outcomes for this cohort of women with breast cancer.

Breast cancer is presented as an example; other cancers in the context of comorbidity must be integrated. It is not known which diseases and other age-related health conditions are present at the time of a cancer diagnosis and to what extent the concomitant conditions compete for care and treatment, nor is there much information on how to treat cancer in the presence of pre-existing chronic conditions. Stronger ties need to be made between geriatric medicine and medical oncology to meet the current and future needs of the older age segment of the population. The demographic and epidemiologic data foretell the expanding U.S. population. The challenge is to understand the multiple clinical and quality care dimensions to meet what an aging population and potentially greater burden of cancer may impose on our health-care system as the number of older persons increases.

Dr. William Robinson, Director, Office of Minority Health and Health Disparities, Health Resources and Services Administration: Dr. Yancik, your study of comorbidity started with age 55, and it looks as though you would have missed quite a bit of information if you had started with age 65.

Dr. Yancik: Thank you for bringing that up. You recall my addressing the heterogeneity of age. In our study, we had a woman in the 55 to 64 age interval who had 10 comorbidities, and that shows that you may have uneven distribution of some of the age-related diseases. I tend to not use the word *elderly* unless I mean it. The demarcation point depends on what we address, but I try to use the terms *older persons* or *older women.*

Dr. Robinson: My point is that we are looking at people in the second half of their lives, and if we were to somehow come up with a term that would pick that up, it might be helpful. We generally choose the 65 year mark because of historical Medicare and Social Security entitlements. Also, for a number of minority people, for people who tend to die a little bit earlier, we lose so many of them in the statistics if we stick with the older intervals.

Dr Yancik: Agreed, often I say that 65 is arbitrary and was chosen because it is our entitlement age, but that was in the 1930s. As you saw from the life expectancy slide, 65 was considered very old in the first part of this century. So we are stuck with the 65 and older definition, but we always have to qualify it.

I should mention that, in the breast cancer study's case, the 55 to 64 interval was added as a comparison group, because this malignancy's incidence tends to rapidly increase in the postmenopausal years. The other six tumors under study—colon, prostate, ovary, bladder, cervix, and stomach data—also include this comparison group.

Dr. Thomas Burish, Provost, Notre Dame University: You have provided a great deal of descriptive data: for example, that cancer is a disease of elderly people, that comorbidity is diagnosed at different stages, and so forth. Now if you had to identify the three biggest problems in cancer in elderly people that are not problems of cancer in younger people, that are unique to this population or much more prominent in this population, that this NCPF might look into or make recommendations about, what would those special challenges be?

Dr. Yancik: Certainly, regarding the "geriatric imperative" and its implications, comorbidity is at the very top on that list of challenges just after the diagnosis of cancer. There is not enough attention to aging and cancer treatment or the research interface. It is worrisome that the normal and pathological processes of aging in combination make it difficult to provide sufficient knowledge on treatment and care for the age group in which cancer primarily occurs. Speaking from a cancer care perspective, focusing on the second part of the title given to me, "implications for medical oncology," is very important. What workforce will be in place to care for older patients with cancer and concurrent health problems? Social support, broadly defined, is a third challenge. Do you have a daughter who can take you to the doctor's appointment or hospital? Do you have a daughter-in-law that can help? Does the patient have grown children? Social support means a caregiver, husband, wife, or friend. The diagnosis of cancer is devastating. Treatment requires support. Survivorship requires assistance.

Ms. Deborah Boyle, Practice Outcomes Nurse Specialist, Banner Good Samaritan Medical Center: I recently heard a geriatrician speaking about the future, the importance of the baby boomers, and that we are the first culture of divorce. He made a projection that a middle-aged woman, married with one child, could divorce and remarry. Her ex-husband could remarry. She could be in her middle 60s and have parents in their 80s. Her one daughter, as she reaches middle age, could be responsible for anywhere from 8 to 12 old people and be expected to provide around-the-clock support in the home with very little training. I think we are only considering the tip of the iceberg of future demands on families and more formal support structures.

Dr. Stephanie Studenski, Professor, Geriatric Medicine, University of Pittsburgh School of Medicine: For me, one of the huge issues is the possibility that the biology of cancer is very different in older people. It seems to be more of a chronic condition, such as prostate cancer and even some breast cancer. I am interested in how we decide on treatment, given very different survival expectations. How do we balance treatment burden and long-term consequences? It seems that too much of the time we take decisions for managing cancer in midlife and apply them to people in late life, even though some of the key factors regarding treatment and consequences may be different.

As another, perhaps irreverent, corollary of that, we worked this summer on a project to understand why fear of breast cancer seems to trump all competing goods. For example, consider hormone replacement and mortality from hip fracture versus breast cancer. Mortality from hip fracture is so much higher than from breast cancer in late life, but we will not give treatments that help hip fracture if they might affect breast cancer risk. We need to rethink how we balance our treatment decisions and perhaps even the way we do clinical trials in light of the biology and natural history of some kinds of cancer in older people. It is not just about survival. It is about the burden of the tumor, the burden of the treatment.

Dr. Yancik: My last comment once again regards the oncology workforce. The American Society of Clinical Oncology (ASCO) has contracted with the Association of American Medical Colleges (AAMC) to look at current medical oncologists in the workforce and the implications of the changing demographics and disease burden on manpower available to provide high-quality care to future cancer patients. This is an important topic to address in a forum with an ASCO and AAMC partnership. I should add that there are some dedicated oncologists who, like Patricia Ganz, have been combining geriatrics and oncology in research and practice for years.

Dr. Barbara Given, Professor of Nursing, Michigan State University: At least for the age groups discussed so far, over 70, if there is not support, we have to worry about the coordination of care. We do not prepare family members to manage all the care that is now outpatient, such as the multiple oral agents and their side effects, compared to years past when the infusions were given in cancer centers.

I think primary care providers get the elderly cancer patient back sooner from the specialty system than some of the younger patients, and the family must worry about coordinating care. I believe that access to home care and support for cancer patients is less, for example, than for COPD or hip fracture. Cancer patients are not necessarily homebound, so they are not eligible for home care, and family members are called on for support. The whole continuum of care, the quality of that care, and the outcomes that are achieved by the formal system depend so much on support that often it must be provided by the family.

Dr. Edward Benz, President, Dana Farber Cancer Institute: The striking information just shown and the question about how this group of patients differs from younger patients suggested to me that we might alert people about updating informal guidelines in various practice communities. I am thinking, for example, of still defining candidacy for prostate cancer surgery, in part, by age over 60. That may be an out-of-date formula based on a cohort of patients that is not relevant to the one we are seeing today. Those patients are choosing options for their therapy based on physician recommendations that might not be appropriate given today's ideas about who is old and who is not.

My other concern is about the clinical trials issue. I was struck by the data regarding stomach cancer. Some 66 percent of patients with stomach cancer are age 65 or older. You overlay that on the list of comorbidities, and it is hard to imagine a stomach cancer patient who would not be ineligible for a clinical trial either explicitly by the criteria or by the medical judgment of the oncologist.

I recall from my early training that a cancer patient could not get a coronary bypass, the belief being they would not live long enough to benefit from it. Today's patients carry labels, like comorbidities, but the physiologic health of people carrying those labels may not be the same as in the past. Shouldn't we look harder at a more functional way of defining these comorbidities and of considering patients for trials?

Dr. Ferrell: When we were planning this workshop, one of the other topics on the table was family caregiving. I want to emphasize the issues raised about the setting of care for older people, in particular home care support. Within the last month, I finished a study that followed 100 lung cancer patients in my cancer center. It was striking to me that instead of following the older patients in the hospital for chemotherapy or serious symptoms as we would have 10 or 20 or more years ago, these older, late-stage patients with serious symptoms and comorbidities, with intensive chemotherapy, surgery, and radiation, most of whom died of their disease, were rarely hospitalized. This is what cancer in elderly people is all about: seriously ill patients being cared for at home by caregivers who may themselves be old or infirm.

Dr. Rebecca Silliman, Professor of Medicine and Public Health, Boston University Schools of Medicine and Public Health: Clinical and Delivery System Issues—Comorbidity and Quality of Care: I will be talking about older cancer patients in general using breast cancer as a model and focusing on screening, early-stage treatment, and surveillance and survivorship, and then I will end with some comments about ways I think we might try to move things forward.

Aging is marked by increased heterogeneity across organ function, comorbidities, functional status, life experiences, and support systems, among others. There is a decreased ability to maintain homeostasis due to decreased functional reserves and impaired compensatory mechanisms. Older patients challenge us, bringing factors such as their aging, their lifelong or recent behaviors, their functional status, and their comorbidities, all influencing in varying degrees their physiology and the clinical encounter. And this is true, by and large, for older patients either with or without cancer. They are similar, perhaps with the exception of patients with cancers that are smoking or alcohol related.

Figure 2-9 displays chronic conditions by age group and emphasizes the important increase in the burden of comorbidity with age, and Table

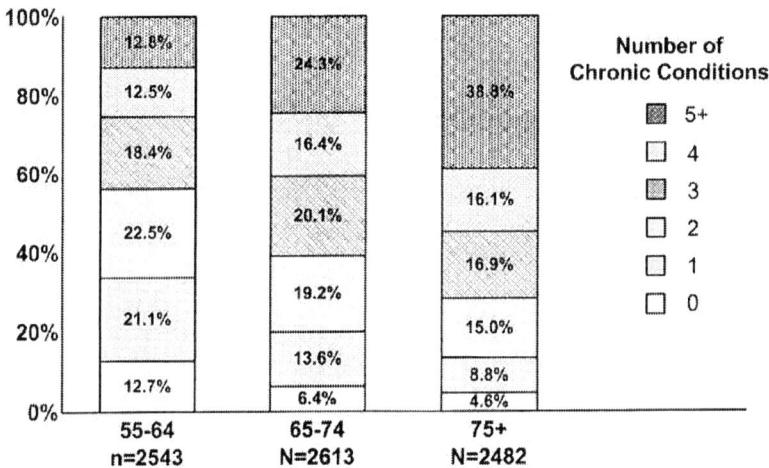

FIGURE 2-9 Number and percent of chronic conditions by age group.
SOURCE: Adapted by Silliman from Yancik, 1997a.

TABLE 2-4 Functional Status in Newly Diagnosed Cancer Patients: New Mexico

Function	65–74 years (%)	75–84 years (%)	85+ years (%)
Bathing	4.4	10.0	24.4
Dressing	4.7	7.4	19.2
Toileting	2.2	4.1	14.1
Transfers	4.7	7.0	16.7
Feeding	1.1	0.7	5.1
Any	7.8	14.1	25.3
Housework	12.6	30.9	65.8
Assistive devices	11.3	20.1	43.6
Transportation	22.8	40.1	68.4
Getting to doctor	4.2	9.7	10.3
Poor memory	27.7	40.4	64.5
Incompetent	2.7	10.0	26.6

SOURCE Adapted by Silliman from Goodwin, 1991.

2-4 lists the declining functional status with age in a group of older cancer patients in New Mexico.

The important thing to note is the increasing challenges focused primarily in the oldest-old in bathing, transfers, toileting, dressing, and other activities related to mobility. Importantly, about 25 percent of people with cancer over the age of 85 have functional disabilities in basic activities of daily living, and this is very similar to figures for noncancer patients. Also particularly important to this audience is the issue of transportation. Certainly, geriatricians would cringe at the word *incompetent*, but here it is a proxy for dementia, and about a quarter of folks over the age of 85 have dementing illnesses (Goodwin et al., 1991).

To move on to screening: we all know that with screening mammography there are few data in this age group to inform what we do. Nonetheless, organizations weigh-in with advice. The American Geriatrics Society recommends that physicians should strongly consider mammography until age 75 with no upper age limit for women with an estimated life expectancy of four more years. The U.S. Preventive Services Task Force recommends screening mammography at age 40 and older, and asserts that the evidence is generalizable to women age 70 and older if their life expectancy is not compromised by comorbid disease. Of course, the challenge is how good physicians are at estimating future life expectancy.

The Breast Cancer in Older Women Research Consortium examined the cost-effectiveness of breast cancer screening taking into account costs, benefits, harms, age, biology, and health status. They found that screening was cost-effective (at $82,000/year of life saved) stopping at age 79 and might be effective beyond that time under certain circumstances, especially for women in the top 25 percent of life expectancy for their age (Mandelblatt et al., 2005). These results were very sensitive to health status, again indicating that comorbidity is the crux of the matter.

Having said this, what do doctors say that they do? In a survey of over 2,000 primary care physicians who responded to scenarios about women ages 70, 80, or 90 at three levels of comorbidity and disability, 31 percent were somewhat or very likely to offer a mammographic screening to a frail, 90-year-old woman with a median life expectancy of 1.8 years, and 79 percent were somewhat or very likely to offer screening to a healthy 80-year-old woman with a median life expectancy of 13 years (Heflin et al., 2006). One could argue that 79 percent is great, but it means that 21 percent of the time a healthy 81-year-old woman would not be offered screening mammography. This illustrates another key issue that is not unique to oncology. In old age, we get it right some of the time, but we also get it wrong a great deal of the time. We get it wrong in two ways: doing too much to those who are too sick and too little for those that are well.

Data on screening mammography in Medicare beneficiaries show what actually happened in 2000–2001. Among those at low risk of death due to comorbidity, 70 percent of what we, in geriatrics, call young-old women ages 65–69 were screened, and 48 percent of those 85 or older were screened. Of those at high risk of death, 19 percent of younger women were screened, and only 5 percent of those 85 or older were screened (Bynum et al., 2005). Again, this illustrates the problem of too little for some, too much for others.

What do we know about tolerance for treatment in older adults? I should note, first of all, that data regarding long-term and late effects of any treatments in older adults are sparse. With respect to surgery, although operative mortality rates are higher and longer-term mortality rates are also higher, there is an important proportion of older persons who enjoy long-term survival following surgical management, and I believe that many of the newer minimally invasive techniques hold great promise of minimizing recovery times in older adults.

With respect to radiation therapy, side effects are no worse in older persons, but their impact may be greater due to associated comorbidities, such as COPD and decreased physiologic reserve as a function of aging. Other treatments, such as surgery and a prolonged prediagnosis phase caused by older people presenting in a very nonspecific way, may make nutritional support more critical and problematic prior to radiation therapy. Further compromising nutrition, radiation may cause decreased salivary gland function, nausea, diarrhea, and malabsorption. Logistical matters such as transportation and osteoporotic, kyphotic, or arthritic backs hindering proper positioning may make radiation therapy difficult at the older ages.

We know that chronological age, per se, is not a particularly strong predictor of chemotherapy toxicity and nonresponse, and from a psychological perspective, many older persons actually tolerate chemotherapy better than their younger counterparts. Newer oral agents and strategies to support patients, such as antiemetics and bone marrow stimulants, are potentially as important if not more important for older than for younger patients. However, people with cancer over age 65 are substantially underrepresented in clinical trials to define these problems and in general. This is particularly true of breast cancer patients: women age 65 or older make up 49 percent of the population with breast cancer, but only 9 percent of those participating in breast cancer clinical trials (Hutchins et al., 1999). Subsequent studies reported somewhat higher proportions of older women in breast cancer trials, but, even if the absolute numbers are increased, this problem of representational bias is huge. So I would encourage you to think about it in your clinical trial discussions. If the trials include only healthy, functional patients without comorbid diseases, practicing physicians will still struggle to generalize and apply trial results to the patient they actually see.

Returning to chemotherapy in elderly people for a moment: certainly, normal aging is associated with increased susceptibility to myelosuppression. Severe, life-threatening neutropenia is more common in older patients, and, obviously, low neutrophil counts can lead to treatment delays, dose reductions, and decreased treatment efficacy. But we can not forget the other potential toxicities involving the heart, the central and peripheral nervous systems, hearing, and the gastrointestinal (GI) tract, all of which can either create or exacerbate existing comorbidities.

So there are three important reasons we should care about comorbidity and functional status in older cancer patients. Cancer therapy may interact with comorbidity to compromise future quality of life through its impact on functional status. Cancer therapy may not affect future life expectancy,

TABLE 2-5 Odds of Nonreceipt of Primary Tumor Therapy for Early-Stage Breast Cancer in Older Women (with 95% Confidence Intervals)

	Nonprimary Therapy	No ALND[a]	No RT[b] After BCS[c]
Age			
65–69	1	1	1
70–74	0.9 (0.6, 1.4)	1.1 (0.8, 1.6)	1.2 (0.7, 2.0)
75–79	2.9 (1.9, 4.3)	3.3 (2.3, 4.9)	4.0 (2.2, 7.0)
80+	5.8 (3.9, 8.6)	8.7 (5.8, 13.2)	11.1 (6.8, 18.2)
Charlson[d]			
0	1	1	1
1–2	1.5 (1.2, 2.0)	1.8 (1.4, 2.3)	1.5 (1.1, 2.0)
3+	2.1 (1.2, 3.8)	3.2 (1.8, 5.6)	1.9 (1.0, 3.6)
Recurrence risk			
Low	2.4 (1.8, 3.4)	2.1 (1.5, 2.8)	1.1 (0.7, 1.6)
Medium	1.6 (1.1, 2.3)	1.8 (1.4, 2.3)	0.8 (0.5, 1.1)
High	1	1	1

[a]ALND = axillary lymph node dissection.
[b]RT = radiotherapy.
[c]BCS = breast-conserving surgery.
[d]Charlson = comorbidity index, proportional to 1-year mortality risk.
SOURCE: Adapted by Silliman from Enger et al., 2006.

because of competing causes of mortality. Cancer therapy may be too risky because of the types and burden of comorbidities and functional impairments. The challenge is to figure out which of these pertain to a given patient.

In spite of our pleas to pay attention to comorbidity and functional status, age has been and remains the strongest independent predictor of receipt of standard cancer treatments. Table 2-5 displays results from a study of 1,859 women 65 and older, with 20 percent in the 80 and older group, who presented with stage I or stage II breast cancer between 1990 and 1994. Although the data show some effects by comorbidities and risk of recurrence (tumor characteristics), the effect of age, particularly being 75 years or older, is strikingly associated with nonstandard primary tumor therapy and failure to receive axillary lymph node dissection and/or radiation therapy after breast-conserving surgery (Enger et al., 2006).

It has been argued that these treatment variations only matter if they

TABLE 2-6 Odds of Breast Cancer Recurrence and Mortality Associated with Less Definitive Care

Variable	Recurrence	Mortality
Prognostic evaluation		
Definitive	1.0	1.0
Less	1.7 (1.0–2.7)	2.2 (1.2–3.9)
Therapy		
Definitive	1.0	1.0
Less	1.6 (1.0–2.6)	1.7 (1.0–2.8)

SOURCE: Adapted by Silliman from Lash et al., 2000.

affect outcomes. Table 2-6 displays the 5-year follow-up of a cohort that colleagues and I assembled and followed in Rhode Island. The data show that nonstandard care is a risk factor for breast cancer recurrence and mortality (Lash et al., 2000). This finding has been replicated more recently using the SEER-Medicare dataset (Smith et al., 2006). In this study, radiation therapy following breast-conserving surgery was associated with a reduced risk of recurrence among older women.

There is another important aspect of the breast cancer story. Given that only about 40,000 of the annual 200,000 incident patients diagnosed with breast cancer die, there is a huge reservoir of prevalent disease in older adults. Even the newest ASCO guidelines on breast cancer follow-up and management are silent on the issue of age and surveillance (Khatcheressian et al., 2006). Again using the SEER-Medicare dataset, Keating and colleagues demonstrated that increasing age is associated with decreased odds of receiving surveillance mammography, even when taking into account demographic and tumor characteristics, comorbidity, and health-care utilization (Keating et al., 2006). Women continuing to visit a cancer specialist and a primary care physician were more likely to receive surveillance mammography. Recent research suggests that patients seen by both a primary care physician and an oncologist also are more likely to receive guideline preventive care for a number of conditions (Earle et al., 2003). Even though there are no clinical trials that have been designed to look at what is recommended for surveillance for older breast cancer patients or for breast cancer patients in general, data from our studies indicate that guideline surveillance is not only associated with a 0.66-fold decrease in the odds of mortality (95 percent confidence interval [CI], 0.50,0.86), but also with a decrease in cancer-related worries (odds ratio [OR] = 0.37, 95 percent CI, 0.14, 0.99) (Lash et al., 2005).

So what are some strategies to improve the care of the older cancer patient? A thoughtful clinical assessment with rationales as follows is an important beginning: to identify risk factors for adverse consequences; to diagnose and treat conditions that put persons at risk for adverse consequences; to prospectively put in place preventive interventions; and, lastly, to guide the choice of therapies and inform patients and families regarding risks and benefits.

The real question is how to do it, and I am not convinced that we, in geriatrics, have come up with the optimal way. The best work appears to me, however, to be under the auspices of the Cancer and Leukemia Group B Cancer in the Elderly Committee (CALGB), which is one of the NCI-sponsored clinical research groups. They have taken the domains of functional status, comorbidity, cognition, psychological function, social support and functioning, and nutrition and have selected and published measures based on these domains being valid, reliable, brief, adaptable for self-administration, and able to prognosticate regarding risk for morbidity and mortality (Hurria et al., 2006). This assessment has only been pilot tested. It takes about 27 minutes for self-administration. I think it will be very important to see how this plays out in more definitive testing. So, in the meantime, what are some other strategies that might be employed?

Figure 2-10 displays future life expectancy at various ages. We use this in both our geriatric oncology and geriatrics training programs to get clinicians thinking about future life expectancy, because, invariably, people underestimate it. The figure shows that at age 85, if you are in the healthy 25 percent with respect to comorbidity and functional status, your future life expectancy, on average, is almost 10 years. Considering the declines with increasing comorbidity within age groups, but also how amazingly long the average future life is, can be useful when assessing older cancer patients. It is also important to estimate the probability of future life expectancy for the individual as that estimate may deviate from the averages shown in Figure 2-10.

A self-administered questionnaire has been developed that takes into account, and assigns scores to, sex, body mass index (BMI), a range of comorbidities and functioning, and age. As total scores mount, so does the percentage predicted to be likely to die within four years (Lee et al., 2006). I think that the assessment of comorbidity and functional status are key to

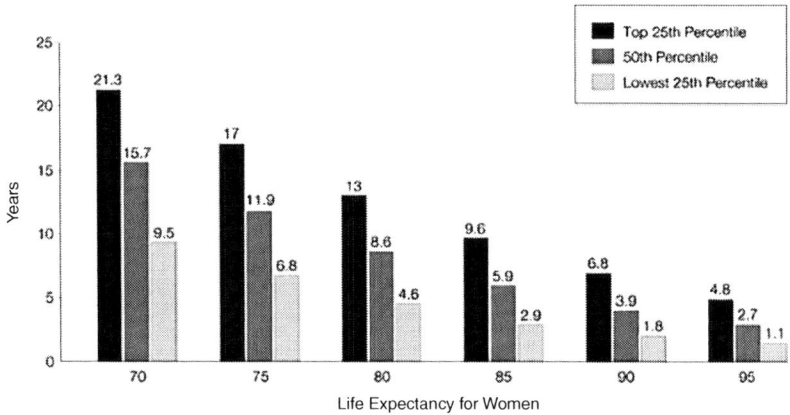

FIGURE 2-10 Life expectancy estimates.
SOURCE Adapted by Silliman from Hurria et al., 2006.

optimal treatment and outcomes for older persons with cancer. The trick, of course, is to figure out how to integrate that into care.

We have much more to learn, and our care systems need to be redesigned to facilitate appropriate assessment and care coordination among primary care providers and cancer specialists for this burgeoning population, particularly its vulnerable subcomponents, of cancer patients.

Dr. Samir Khleif, Food and Drug Administration: I see that assessment of comorbidity is going to be very important, but looking at the percentages of the older patients that participate in clinical trials, I see also a bias that is going to make it difficult to gather new data. Is the solution just to design clinical trials for elderly people, or are there other ways to approach this problem?

Dr. Silliman: I think the design of clinical trials is only part of the answer. Nevertheless, the problem now is that there are either errors introduced by generalizing from clinical trials involving only younger people, or this evidence that is perceived to be nonrepresentational may simply be ignored. But in the future, as more targeted therapies or more oral agents are introduced, there should be opportunities, as was suggested earlier, to involve more heterogeneous populations in clinical trials.

Still, I think there will never be enough clinical trials; therefore, I want better assessments so that age is not the end of the analysis. We should drill down below age and get at the factors that are really problematic for understanding cost and benefit, risks and benefit, comorbidity, functional status, and underlying physiology, among others.

Dr. Edith Perez, Director, Cancer Clinical Study Unit, Mayo Clinic: I remember getting NCI reviews about paying attention to older women. Then we designed trials to include older patients, and NCI asked why specify older women? Why should they be different? So we stopped. Some of the major problems have been discussed. First, there is a perception by physicians that older patients have low life expectancy and have already lived their lives. Patients often seem to agree that they have lived their lives, and they do not want to be part of a trial with repeated visits, requirements for tissue samples, and the other extra steps.

I think the increasing distance between family-practice residencies and oncology-specialty care means that when patients return to their primary care physician from an oncologic consultation, the primary care provider may consider age and recommend against adjuvant therapy or the like.

I hope it is a solvable problem, but I think it will require that these older patients understand that there is an issue and raise their voices, because if it does not come from them, I do not know how we are going to fix it.

Dr. Stephanie Studenski: As somewhat of an outsider, my perception is that a fundamental goal of many clinical trials is to examine the effect of an agent on a tumor. That is a very important goal, but it may mean the elimination of distracting influences. Can we perform clinical trials that are aligned with the goals of treatment—sometimes it might be eradication of the tumor or a cure—but couldn't we also do trials that examine which of several dosage-adjustment protocols or agent choices give the longest independent functioning or something to that effect?

To me, one of the issues is the way the question is set up. It may not be the best thing to accrue my group to your trials, but they do have clinical questions important to answer and could be rigorously studied. I worry that, to the extent that a great deal of the funding is in partnership with the private sector, the motivation may be mostly to generate new products through clean studies. I have been trying to think how to motivate the private sector to want an evidence base for how to use their preferred drugs for the great variety of cancers and situations that one sees in the real world—in other words, to increase clinical trial participation in older people by designing trials that are not age limited but that have a focus on different clinical goals.

Dr. Jerome Yates, Director of Research, American Cancer Society: In the early 1970s when we were treating acute myelogenous leukemia, we found that we could ablate the bone marrow, but the older people did much worse than the younger age groups. Some said this was because of inadequate supportive care, but it is probably resistant disease because of the karyotypes that we know persist in the older population. Nevertheless, I also received many calls from community physicians who embarked on this therapy in older patients without having adequate supportive care.

We need to provide good supportive care for aggressive therapies, but we also need to be sure that we are not dealing with resistant disease in a particular population. This is probably relevant now to non-Hodgkin's lymphoma. Also, the bulk of the cancers in older people are amenable to surgical cure, if we can discover them early. So the ability to screen the patients becomes very critical as well.

I would also comment that the average community physician does not like to be consulted and then treat the patient and have the patient die. They will treat a 50-year-old outpatient with chemotherapy or aggressive radiotherapy right into the ground. But if you give them a 70-year-old patient, they will be timid and not do the same sort of thing, because they are in a hospital, dependent on referrals, and it is not good for your track record to have your patients die.

Dr. Ganz: Inclusion of representative patients in well-designed clinical trials is important for advancing science and the delivery of care, but for many of the common diseases that we see in elderly people, it is surgery, radiation, and screening that are important. It may be hormonal therapies in both breast and prostate cancer. These patients often have localized disease, and for them we do not necessarily need more clinical trials. We just need the appropriate dissemination and delivery of standard care, which I think we determined 20 years ago in our various studies.

Most people with colon cancer are operated on. There is no question about that. They may not get adjuvant therapy, which, I think, is a dissemination issue. Most women with a lump in the breast will have it removed, but they may not get the radiation to the breast that will prevent the recurrence, which will be much more morbid to treat five or six years later when that woman is older. So I think we need to insist on standard quality of care, both with screening and early detection where there are evidence and appropriate age guidances, and standard delivery of these kinds of care. I think it is appalling that a woman with a lump in her breast who did not get radiation does not get subsequent mammography. This is unacceptable and intolerable, and this is the policy issue.

I think as we baby boomers move into older age, we are going to be different consumers. We are not going to be as complacent, and the demography of aging will change as a result of this, because we have faced our health-care differently. But I think there are very important policy implications about just delivering what we know works, not using age as the criterion, but using some other method to say this is justifiable treatment.

Dr. Khleif: But don't you think that this is a catch-22 in a way? Because if standard therapy is being determined by clinical trials, and if clinical trials are biased toward younger populations, there will be a bias built into delivering standard care.

Dr. Ganz: But we are talking about surgery and radiation, where we have consensus conference guidelines. There is no age dictum. There have been many trials focused on the need for breast radiation in older women. One might find maybe a sub-subgroup that you can just treat with endocrine therapy with lumpectomy, but, by and large, they all need radiation, and there have been some targeted trials looking at older women. We are talking about management strategies where for many tumors, such as prostate cancer and colon cancer, there have been good overviews of the clinical trials data in elderly people who did participate, and they do tolerate adjuvant therapy. Lower representation of older patients in trials still does not explain why there isn't dissemination of adjuvant therapy in stage III colon cancer.

Dr. Silliman: There still seems to be this notion that people are going to die of something else before they die of their cancer, ergo, if we just give them a little bit of therapy, then everything will be fine. What I have tried to do is provide as solid evidence as I can that that is a very bad idea.

Dr. Kathleen Foley, Attending Neurologist, Memorial Sloan-Kettering Cancer Center: There are some models suggesting how to perform clinical trials in this population that relate to linking phase 1 trials to patients who are also candidates for hospice care. They are given support through palliative care or a hospice situation at the same time they are participating in a phase 1 trial. There is a demonstration project that looks quite successful, and, at least at M.D. Anderson Cancer Center, the phase 1 trial group is closely aligned with the palliative and hospice care group. So the patients who move into that phase 1 trial, because there is nothing else available, readily become candidates and have a continuity of care model that is effective. That is one thought.

There is a second thought. A recent review of Medicare data in Massachusetts and California examined the use of chemotherapy in patients in the last 6, 3, and 1 month of life. In this group of patients, age 65 or older, 23–33 percent received chemotherapy in the last 6 months of life and 9 percent in the last month. The tumor's responsiveness to chemotherapy did not seem to influence whether dying patients received this treatment at the end of life (Emanuel et al., 2003).

This study suggests to me the possibility, from a cost-effective perspective, that patients who move to a third-line or fourth-line therapy should be part of a clinical trial, and that would, in a way, engage us to take on an elderly population, since, for the most part, those are the groups that are in that population. I think there is an opportunity from a policy perspective to think about linking and bridging palliative care with phase 1 trials. Of course, there is also the policy question of oncologists giving ineffective therapies that waste Medicare funds just because they feel they have to do something for a patient, and it is clearly the patients older than 65 years for which we have the data.

Ms. Boyle: I think Dr. Khleif is correct in terms of looking at this issue of ageism and bias. We would not automatically assume that young children could tolerate the same type of chemotherapy as a 30-year-old, given the differences in pharmacokinetics and pharmacodynamics. We have a very at-risk population here, because of comorbidity, because of different handling of drugs, and because of the likelihood of polypharmacy. And so, even if we look at physiological rather than chronological age in terms of their eligibility for clinical trials, because of these factors many elderly people will be automatically excluded. The real result, then, is that there is no standard way to measure what is the best combination of drugs for this population. Maybe there are some drugs that are less toxic, for a variety of reasons, that could be substituted, but if older patients do not participate in clinical trials, we are left with conjecture or past experience. Yet, these are the majority of people who have cancer, and my view is that we are treating the majority of people who have cancer with drug regimens that have not been tested in this group. I can not think of another indication in cancer care where that happens.

So the handful of physicians in the United States that are looking at geriatric oncology suggest that we look at three subsets of patients: the very fit—physiologically, chronologically, and so on; those who are in the middle with some comorbidity and chronic illness, but not frail; and those who are very frail, what people think of as elderly, in the rocking chair in the nursing home. I think, however, that this shows our bias, because we would never do that with children. We would automatically look at them very individually.

Dr. Robinson: In defense of some of my comrades in primary care, we are trying to handle each patient as an individual, and there is no single population-wide standard of care. The negative outcome to the patient is one thing. The physician's reputation is one thing. They are also trying to practice good medicine, and the problem may be the lack of dialogue between the oncologists who have a sense of what could or should be done and the primary care practitioners approaching the cancer system uncertain about what to do. Patients are caught between the person they are relying on for all of their comorbid conditions or their primary care, if they are still in good health, and the person caring for their new and serious problem with cancer.

In the past, the Food and Drug Administration (FDA) demanded that there be uniformity in all of the patients in clinical trials for ease in analyzing the data, even though we know that the drugs were going to be prescribed for people who were anything but the ideal persons in the trials. So that FDA argument still has to be put on the table, and they need to be a part of a solution.

Dr. Yates: I see three issues. One is the condition of the patient, the second is the treatment, and the third is your ability to support that patient through the problems created by the treatment. When we developed guidelines with the National Comprehensive Cancer Network for elderly people, one of the first things to come up was the discomfort of the oncologist in dealing with the older patients. So the geriatricians there suggested that these patients ought to be seen by a geriatrician before embarking on some of the aggressive treatments. Then, we polled the people at the table whether or not they had geriatricians on their staff, and about half of them did, but they said it would take two weeks to get a geriatric consult. So it was impractical.

Maybe the short-term solutions such as the CALGB patient assessment will provide us with some of the answers, but the question of how aggressive you get in terms of life-threatening treatments is really difficult. Surgery is a little easier, because we can carry most people for a week or so.

Dr. Khleif: We have taken a number of steps, such as geriatric oncology and committees or consortia for older cancer patients, and now I am wondering if there are options beside clinical trials specifically for older persons?

Dr. Silliman: I have performed observational studies all of my life. They certainly have their challenges, and there are some that will not consider evidence from an observational study to be valid, but I think if such studies are carefully performed they can provide useful information. We need all the evidence we can get, and it can not all be just clinical trial evidence for all the reasons that we have talked about. We can not rely on clinical trials or else it will be 2030 and we will be having this conversation one more time.

Dr. Studenski: Disability, either transient or persistent, related to cancer and its treatment is common but the evidence base is painfully thin and has not been a research priority. Research on cancer-related disability could be incorporated into ongoing human studies. Cancer and cancer treatment affect function in ways that were not anticipated when treatments were developed. We can anticipate that many cancers and their treatments will affect disability, and so we should plan care around assessment and monitoring of function as well as cancer response. There are collaborative ways to intervene on disability with cancer. Cancer in older people is emerging as a longer-term, more chronic condition than an acute condition, and we need to incorporate disability into decision making about the way we think about and care for cancer.

We do not need to compete for research concerns and priorities. Both a biomedical perspective and a functional perspective promote good science and good patient care. Remember that consumers, patients, and families experience illness as symptoms and effects on function, not biomarkers or abnormal lab tests. We, as providers, can integrate biomedical thinking with symptoms and function. The practice of geriatrics may be considered an integrated approach to pathophysiologic processes as they affect symptoms and function.

How does cancer disable older people? Cancer can damage organ systems, such as the brain or bone, leading to dysfunction and disability. Disability can result from cancer's systemic effects such as fatigue and pain. Cancer treatments can cause disability through such systemic effects as fatigue or through more specific consequences such as malnutrition or neuropathy. In the older cancer patient, cancer and cancer treatment interact a great deal with prior disease and disability. Vulnerability to disability with cancer and cancer treatment is affected by functional status prior to treatment.

Our understanding of disability in the older cancer patient is strongly affected by the current approach to obtaining evidence. There are important selection factors at every point in the accrual of data. For a person to become a source of directly obtained data, they must be referred for cancer care (and there may be a very frail population that never gets diagnosed or referred), and then referred to an academic center that participates in research, and then finally recruited to a study. We get our data in two main ways. We can use administrative datasets, which are wonderful, because they capture a broad population without individual volunteers. These data are more generalizable, but most such datasets lack information on function. Datasets based on Medicare lack information on functional status. A short functional status scale for use in Medicare could open up opportunity for cancer researchers if it could be included more broadly. Directly collected data can include function, but data based in directly recruited patient samples are much less representative and generalizable. In summary, our evidence base about cancer and function in older adults is often skewed and is only the tip of the iceberg.

What do we know? Figure 2-11 displays odds ratios for associations between cancer survival status and functional limitations in Medicare beneficiary female cancer survivors of median age 72 years. These are 5-year cancer survivors' burden of disability across a range of cancers, adjusted for other factors that contribute to disability. Women without cancer are the comparison group. Women with many kinds of cancer have much higher odds of disability 5 years later (Sweeney et al., 2006). It is still not clear if the disability is a consequence of the cancer or cancer treatment or if there

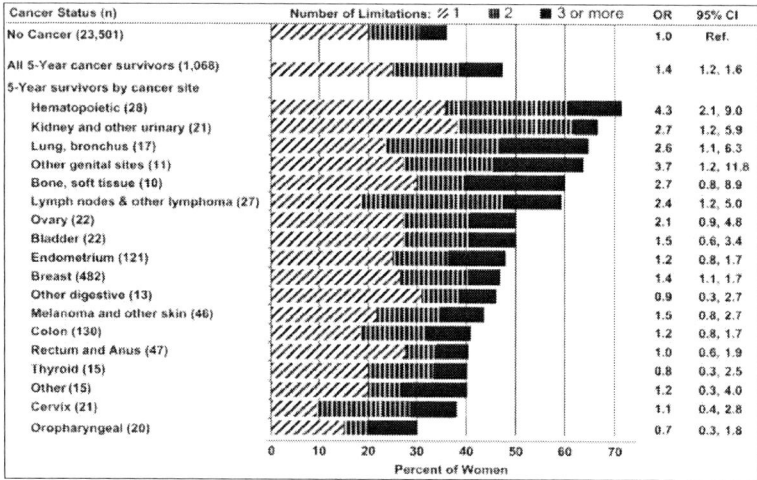

Cancer Status (n)	Number of Limitations: ⁄ 1 █ 2 ■ 3 or more	OR	95% CI
No Cancer (23,501)		1.0	Ref.
All 5-Year cancer survivors (1,068)		1.4	1.2, 1.6
5-Year survivors by cancer site			
Hematopoietic (28)		4.3	2.1, 9.0
Kidney and other urinary (21)		2.7	1.2, 5.9
Lung, bronchus (17)		2.6	1.1, 6.3
Other genital sites (11)		3.7	1.2, 11.8
Bone, soft tissue (10)		2.7	0.8, 8.9
Lymph nodes & other lymphoma (27)		2.4	1.2, 5.0
Ovary (22)		2.1	0.9, 4.8
Bladder (22)		1.5	0.6, 3.4
Endometrium (121)		1.2	0.8, 1.7
Breast (482)		1.4	1.1, 1.7
Other digestive (13)		0.9	0.3, 2.7
Melanoma and other skin (46)		1.5	0.8, 2.7
Colon (130)		1.2	0.8, 1.7
Rectum and Anus (47)		1.0	0.6, 1.9
Thyroid (15)		0.8	0.3, 2.5
Other (15)		1.2	0.3, 4.0
Cervix (21)		1.1	0.4, 2.8
Oropharyngeal (20)		0.7	0.3, 1.8

Percent of Women

FIGURE 2-11 Disability in 5-year cancer survivors.
NOTE: Odds ratios are adjusted for demographics, health, and comorbid conditions.
SOURCE: Adapted by Studenski from Sweeney et al., 2006.

are other uncontrolled factors associated with being a cancer survivor that increase the likelihood of disability.

What do we know about treatment effects on disability? In one observational study of patients age 65 years or older with breast, lung, prostate, or colon cancer who were assessed using SF-36 (a 36-item short form health survey) scores, patients were compared with national norms for ages 55–64 immediately before a cancer diagnosis and at 6 to 8 weeks after diagnosis. The data confirm that older cancer patients referred for cancer care are a select group. The cancer patients in this study had better health and function scores before diagnosis of breast, prostate, or colon cancer diagnosis than the national norms, but the scores declined to (prostate cancer) or below (breast, lung, and colon cancer) national norms at 6 to 8 weeks. These losses in functioning were related to treatment, not comorbidities (Given et al., 2001).

Censoring of data across the duration of the clinical study can bias findings about function and health status. In a study of disability in a cervical cancer clinical trial, several function and health status measures were administered prior to randomization and over 1 year of chemotherapy and follow-up. Scores were generally stable over time and considerably better than general population norms (McQuellon et al., 2006). But the effects of censoring may have influenced the findings. The study began with about 250 participants and ended with about 140. Over half the survivors did not complete the final surveys. These survivors who did not complete surveys had worse health and function scores at earlier assessments. Therefore, a major problem with self-report of function is that data may be lost among participants who are not doing well. The censoring is directional; patients with good quality of life are more likely to remain respondents. The actual burden of disability may be much higher if the effects of censoring are considered.

How should we measure disability? The field offers numerous measures, diverse terminology, and variable conceptual frameworks. Quality of life, physical function, and functional performance can be considered similar constructs by some but very distinct by others. Subjective and objective measures differ in perspective and sometimes in reliability. There are also limits to how much time and inconvenience people will tolerate to complete questionnaires. Since bias can develop from those who get sick and do not complete surveys. We need to develop reliable data sources from proxy respondents.

The use of disability assessment should differ based on a range of planned uses, such as screening, classification, measuring change, and treatment planning. For screening, the goal should be to eliminate subjects that do not require any more survey time. For example, high-functioning people who do not have any disability do not need to be asked in detail about bathing and dressing. For classification, we need an instrument that is short and quite coarse, a type of performance status indicator that sorts people into large groups and is useful for initial triage. For measuring change, transient disability is common and clinically important, and the preferred instrument should be sensitive enough to detect it. We should also be able to monitor recovery of function and persistent disability in the cancer survivor. Such a measure must be sensitive to small but important change and also feasible with proxy respondents, since the more disabled cancer patients are less likely to respond for themselves. Finally, detailed measures of disability are needed for treatment planning. The occupational therapist may need to assess multiple aspects of bathing and dressing in detail, because rehabilitation interventions require a degree of specificity that the rest of us may not need to know. There is no single perfect disability measure, and there should not be.

Some simple performance measures of function can be useful. For ex-

ample, changes in gait speed detect changes in cardiopulmonary, neuro-
logic, and musculoskeletal status. Gait speed may be a powerful global indicator of physiologic reserve and health. When comparing gait speed to
oncologists' assessment of performance status, it is clear that oncologists are
able to classify high-functioning older people who have fast gait speed as
electrocorticography (ECOG) performance status (PS) 0 and lower-func-
tioning older people with slow gait speed as PS 2. They have the most
trouble differentiating among those in the middle, often rated as PS 1,
where the range of gait speed and function can be quite broad. A simple
screening tool such as gait speed might help the oncologist sort out functional groups. They can be reassured about the health of the patients with
PS 0 and perhaps refer the patients with PS 2 for restorative services.
Oncologists need the most help with further evaluation of the PS 1s.

   Life expectancy is at the heart of cancer treatment, but actually it is
about more than survival. In aging, we use the concept of active life expectancy, or expected years of independent functioning. Overall life expectancy
can be divided into years of active and years of restricted functioning. This
concept can be important to older adults and families. Geriatrics as a field
is dedicated to increasing the duration of active life expectancy.

   In a recent study, I applied concepts about active life expectancy to the
way we look at older patient's experience with cancer and cancer treatment.
I used simple measures of number of days spent in bed and number of days
unable to get out of the house as an alternative way to describe the cancer
treatment experience. For example, consider a new treatment that prolongs
survival. If bed days and restricted activity days were monitored, we could
determine the functional cost of the survival gain. If the gain in survival
days is less than the increase in bed days, then the number of functionally
independent days has actually decreased and active life expectancy has decreased. When making treatment decisions, some patients and doctors
might welcome information such as this about the consequences of treatment for function as well as survival. Some people might still choose the
life-prolonging treatment, but they would do so in a way that informs
them of the functional consequences.

   What if the treatment goal is to improve treatment tolerance? A new
treatment might not increase overall survival, but instead it might reduce
bed days and restricted activity days. Perhaps improved active life expectancy could be used to develop or target treatments that emphasize treatment tolerance for older people.

   Bed days and restricted activity days are just another way to measure function. They tap into similar concepts as activities of daily living or many aspects of quality of life. They may offer an interpretable metric for patients and providers because bed days are within lay experience. Patients can imagine days spent in bed and relate them to their own lives. One limitation of current quality of life and function scales is that, while developed with elegant psychometrics, they are often opaque and hard to interpret for most of us. The scales yield a number that does not have intrinsic meaning to patients' families and providers. Numbers of days in bed or days unable to leave the house may have intrinsic meaning to most of us, because that is the way we talk: "He was sick; he was in bed all week." This familiarity from everyday experience can be used to create accessible and interpretable measure of function.

Peripheral neuropathy is an increasingly common complication of some of the cancer treatments that can result in disability. We do not have consensus on how to detect neuropathy or when to alter treatment because of it, but it is an emerging important issue. A recent study of peripheral neuropathy in ovarian cancer patients in remission after initial chemotherapy (carboplatin and paclitaxel) examined incidence, type, and severity during therapy and at intervals up to and beyond 6 months after treatment. This study went beyond usual event reporting and carefully monitored for neuropathy. The researchers discovered 65 of 120 patients (54 percent) had sensory neuropathy during treatment (three with motor neuropathy as well). Data were available for 60 patients at follow-up, and 14 of those (23 percent) had residual neuropathy after a median follow-up of 18 months. Neuropathy persisted in 9 patients (15 percent) after 6 months. There were some cases of grade 3 neuropathy, which could be expected to have a significant effect on function (Pignato et al., 2006).

We know little about risk or functional consequences of treatment-related neuropathy. We do know that dose and duration of drug exposure are important. Pre-existing peripheral neuropathy may be a predisposing factor. In my clinical experience, 30 or 40 percent of the general population of 70-year-old people will have undetected subclinical peripheral neuropathy, but there are no explicit studies on the subject. There is minimal evidence about how cancer treatment-related neuropathy affects function. There are clinical case reports of people with numb hands and have trouble with buttons and zippers or who have numb feet and become unsteady. Prevention of neuropathy is an important emerging area of study. Trials in these areas should include function and disability as outcomes, not just nerve conduction velocity.

Treatment can affect function and disability in unanticipated ways. Androgen deprivation for prostate cancer can be a long-term treatment with recently recognized functional consequences. Androgen deprivation alters body composition. One recent report describes a 3.8 percent decrease in lean mass (muscle) and an 11 percent increase in fat mass among 79 men with nonmetastatic prostate cancer at 48 weeks after beginning androgen deprivation (Smith, 2004). Such loss of muscle mass and increase in fat mass can affect function. Prostate cancer patients on androgen deprivation have been shown to have significant decrements in quality of life measures compared to those not so treated (Dacal et al., 2006).

Many treatments for cancer were developed when cancer was considered much more of a lethal acute illness. Long-term side effects and their potential for meaningful implications for function were secondary considerations. Treatment is now sometimes chronic and increasingly exposes patients to long-term adverse effects. We need to rethink our decision making about the balance of treatment benefits and harms as we move beyond survival to short- and long-term effects on function as primary inputs into our decision making.

What does rehabilitation offer the cancer patient? Standard treatment includes therapeutic exercise through physical therapy; adaptive equipment and environments; modified self-care strategies provided by occupational therapists; caregiver training; nonpharmacologic pain management; and management of dysphagia. Rehabilitation is not necessarily limited to people with a permanent disability. Rehabilitation can play a role in improving tolerance to treatment, adapting to disability, even in transient disability that may last only a few months, and in helping people with end-of-life care.

There are studies on exercise during and after cancer. Most are small, and many only focus on patients who have completed treatment, but studies during cancer treatment are beginning. So far the effects have been modest. Recent reviews summarize the effects of exercise in cancer patients and the benefits of lifestyle interventions to improve dietary and physical activity behaviors in cancer patients (Knols et al., 2005; Demark-Wahnfried et al., 2006).

Combined interventions that incorporate medications with rehabilitation may be effective and should be tested. For example, functional status end points could be assessed in prostate cancer patients on androgen blockage who are assessed in a clinical trial of agents that reduce loss of muscle mass plus exercise. Elements of exercise or rehabilitation could be tested for ability to contribute to better treatment tolerance and perhaps increased ability to complete a course of therapy. Rehabilitation and exercise could be assessed for ability to promote resilience as a preventive strategy to reduce adverse events. There is almost no evidence base for the efficacy of rehabilitation in geriatric cancer care. It may have potential to prevent, reduce, or promote recovery of disability in combination with thoughtful cancer-treatment planning.

As we select these interventions, we should be thinking about monitoring for peripheral neuropathy if we are going to induce body composition changes. We are going to combine preventive interventions with rehabilitation therapy and help people cope with transient or persistent problems as they develop. Often, we are thinking about such adverse events as neutropenia, but we may not be tracking other important things that are emerging, such as body composition changes as well as neuropathy and its effects on independent function. If we are causing these problems, we should track and intervene in combined ways. I hope, as we move toward keeping cancer patients alive longer and dealing with cancers that seem to smolder for a long time, that we think of disability as an important element for treatment consequences.

Dr. Ferrell: I want to emphasize how important the information you shared about bed days is, because it is so common that older people are presented treatment options and then sons and daughters, well intended, go home thinking that if we start mom on this treatment, we might get two or three months of life with her lung cancer. But they are not thinking about bed days, and this becomes the quality-of-care issue for older people. This morning, we spent a great deal of time talking about older people needing greater access to care, but I hope that our report and this day also captures the significant issue of older people who should not be treated with chemotherapy, because we do a great deal of harm to this group.

At the end of your presentation, you emphasized rehabilitation during the course of treatment, but you also acknowledged, even if active chemotherapy or a trial is decided against, that the care plan at home for many older patients should consider the great benefit of a nutrition consult, of pain management, symptom relief, supportive care, and, then, transition into hospice, and I want to emphasize that your concept of rehabilitation applies outside of active treatment.

Dr. Studenski: The policy problem is that for Medicare reimbursement, you have to have some goal of rehabilitation treatment that involves making people better, but in this kind of situation, many times what you are trying to do is to help people cope, while the culture of rehabilitation is largely focused on improving function.

Dr. Perez: I am concerned about comments implying that we are hurting older patients by treating them. I would caution that we may, potentially, be hurting many people because they are not getting treatment, because they never have access to a discussion about the potential benefits of therapy.

Dr. Ferrell: I agree that it can be both. There is a very significant segment of the older patient population who are being harmed because they do not have access to treatment and trials, but I think it would be an injustice not to recognize that there are significant numbers of older people whose quality of life is probably diminished because they are getting treatments that will not offer much benefit to them.

Dr. Studenski: I think Dr. Silliman was very clear that the problem is that chronologic age is a poor proxy for who is going to benefit and what kind of harms will be done. We need to use other measures of physiologic age. But in addition, even those that are treated appropriately can have consequences of treatment such as transient or persistent disability, and we should be interested in supporting them with appropriate rehabilitation interventions.

Dr. Ganz: You point out that the rehabilitation model is an acute care model. However, we know that we are dealing with many chronic diseases—diabetes or heart failure or cancer—where patients may want to maintain their function rather than to decline. My concerns are how do we change the rehabilitation community, which does not like to deal with these patient populations, and how do we change reimbursement policy so that maintenance of function, keeping somebody independently functioning at home and deferring an assisted-living situation, can be an accepted goal?

Dr. Studenski: I think the big problem is the potential for an open-ended commitment to reimburse for maintenance of health on everybody. I think much of what we call rehabilitation does not necessarily require advanced medical rehabilitation therapy training and involves exercise programs and health behaviors that are not so very complex.

Dr. Ganz: Agreed, yet I just had a discussion with a young male breast-cancer survivor who needs to lose weight, and his wife asked why will our insurance company reimburse bariatric surgery, but a supervised weight-loss program will not be reimbursed? This is the distortion. These interventions can be low-cost and low-tech, maybe just a supervised exercise group of some sort that is much less expensive than having a therapist. If we do not start to think about the needs of the aging and chronic-illness populations then we will not have very rational strategies.

Ms. Deborah Boyle, Nursing Roles and Capacity: When you think about the word *capacity*, think of the competence, the efficiency, the magnitude, and the scope of what nurses can provide to this special population. Although the term implies optimum interventions, it also is indicative of the vulnerability of these patients and the absence of care that many of them need.

We know that nurses and physicians will play different roles in addressing their needs. As George Will wrote in *Newsweek*, "Physicians are an episodic presence in the lives of patients. Nurses control the environment of healing." I think this is because nurses have a central position as choreographer of all the care that the patient receives and as someone who is there around the clock in the inpatient setting and even often in the ambulatory setting. We can be proud that the Oncology Nursing Society has stepped forward for many vulnerable populations, and I certainly think that older people are one of these vulnerable populations. We did so for the needs of cancer survivors, and we wrote our first position paper on cancer in elderly people in 1992 and did a second edit of that paper as a joint position statement in concert with the Geriatric Oncology Consortium in 2004 (Oncology Nursing Society and Geriatric Oncology Consortium, 2004).

Major themes of that joint position paper included the prominent role of ageism as something that must be dealt with in overcoming current barriers; education of current practitioners and students; looking at possibilities of measurement beyond chronologic age and at risks related to declining functional reserve; redefining outcomes beyond disease-free survival to encompass functional status and quality of life; access to care along the cancer trajectory; using interdisciplinary teams and the comprehensive geriatric assessment; provision of specialized care across settings to extended care facilities or assisted living; increased funding that is required based on the prominence of this problem; providing outreach and encouraging clinical trial participation; and, last, but certainly not least, the issue of advocacy and policy in terms of legislation.

I think that there are six major areas of capacity for nurses that work with cancer patients: community awareness, family advocacy, polypharmacy, symptom distress, survivorship, and end-of-life care. When I think of community awareness, as an advocate on the needs of elderly people for probably close to three decades, I ask who is doing anything specific to inform elderly people of their significant age-dependent risk of developing cancer. I have yet to find a specific community intervention that tells them the percentage of people their age that will develop cancer and integrates age-specific sequelae into program design, things such as neurosensory compromise—vision, hearing, and tactile changes that influence self-care and memory.

This is a key role for nurses, because, for many older patients, nurses are seen as very credible experts who see what happens to the patients and are listened to. We must integrate these age-specific sequelae into the programmatic design to let people know they are at heightened risk. This is true whether it is vision, hearing, or tactile change, as I mentioned, or mobility issues, somebody with bad arthritis, kyphosis, or even asking patients to take on self-care and change dressings or learn how to maneuver an ostomy. We fail to acknowledge some of the critical barriers that affect many of our older patients. Certainly memory is a serious issue. Think how you took a very ill child to the doctor's office, and, because of your anxiety, you only remembered a third of what you were told. Consider now our older patients for whom there may be some decline in memory to begin with, and they are told they have a life-threatening illness. They may be there by themselves or have a spouse who also has a similar compromise. We need to be sensitive to these situations, perhaps take some sensitivity training as is provided in gerontology programs.

The other thing, I think, that is critically involved with educating many at-risk older patients is the fatalism that comes with some of the experience they may have had of deaths of people in their social network or a spouse. We tell a patient that she has a very curable breast malignancy, but all she can remember is that her husband had cancer and was dead in 6 weeks. We can not assume that the older patient can make the distinction between acute leukemia and early stage breast cancer.

We should think about the mobility and transportation issues too.

Rarely do *we* go to the older person. We expect them to come to *us*, but there is a reason why the older person asks not to have an appointment after four. It may be a problem with getting about when it is dark, for example. So we should think about taking the message out to the people, rather than having them come to where we are.

We also note that the current elderly population grew up in an era where there was an aversion to medical institutions and physicians—that you only went to the doctor to die. That will not be the case with baby boomers. They will be more assertive and want to make their own decisions. But today, family and the social network as information brokers are key. We know from the patient education literature that if you want to talk to any of the males in the family about prostate cancer or HIV or whatever, you should direct your information to the mothers, and it is their job, as information brokers, to disseminate that information to the rest of the family.

Similarly, with elderly people, especially those with neurosensory compromise, it is important to ask that they bring someone with them when they come in for their consultation. Some progressive medical oncology practices offer to tape the consultation and send it to the daughter back home so that she is not hearing everything second or third hand and has a good understanding of what is going on with her parent.

Last, but certainly not least, is the issue of culture. If the older person has a strong ethnic connection, perhaps as an immigrant, it is very important that we know what those norms are. When we transmit information, who tells it? Who hears it? There may be, for example, the phenomenon of filial piety with many Asian cultures that very directly affects what we do and what we can say to many of our patients.

You will hear more about family advocacy from Dr. Given. However, this is critical. There are many issues that confront patients and families and also frustrate those of us on the front line in terms of providing care. I mentioned earlier that a spouse or other family member who provides around-the-clock care is expected to not only hear what is told them, but be able to synthesize it and know what to do in an emergent situation. This is in addition to the physical burden.

Cognitive dysfunction is one of the biggest deterrents to sending older cancer patients home and expecting a family to keep them at home. Much of these patients' delirium is caused by things that either we do to them or a metabolic problem. But, in addition, there are the physical implications of insomnia, of getting up and helping the husband to the bathroom every half hour, and certainly there are the emotional ramifications for spouses that have been married 40, 50, or 60 years and cannot even begin to anticipate what their life might be like without that partner.

There are also social implications for those older couples that are very socially inclined. And there are informational implications, particularly for the well spouse explaining to the family why X was done versus Y. They are often the liaison with the medical team. Think about how many physicians, office personnel, diagnostic personnel, and pharmacists they are dealing with. There is also the liaison with their external support network that will have questions and recommendations. The hovering nature of many of these family caregivers can be absolutely all consuming.

Although we often think that, by virtue of being old, there are not as many people in a person's social support network, it may be just the opposite. We have to look beyond not just the spouses; there may be elder siblings, adult children, grandchildren, nieces and nephews who think of their uncle as their surrogate father, and nonblood relatives who actually function as family. Then, we have special considerations—what we refer to as the hidden patient. These are the well spouses who have to prepare the food and provide other support. Although we think of them as well, they may have their own medical problems that interfere with their ability to provide care.

I mentioned filial piety as an issue. We also are seeing more and more spouses diagnosed at the same time. And many older patients may have limited family or limited family where they reside to help provide care. This is the sandwich generation, the long-distance children who care very much about their parents, but cannot take up and leave and go to Florida because they have their own husband and children that they care for. And there may be significant cumulative loss. We see so many older patients who have just lost a sibling or a best friend, and now they face their own illness or their spouse's.

On the other hand, those older patients who do well and are sitting in their oncology clinic observing dismal cases of children with terrible cancers will talk about feeling guilty that they are doing so well, when many of the younger patients are not doing as well.

Polypharmacy is certainly one of my particular interests. When we talk about comorbidity, we must talk about polypharmacy. On the average, for every chronic illness that an older person has, they are given at least one to two prescriptions. Although, we think of polypharmacy and prescription drugs, we need to acknowledge that older Americans, again, who represent only 12 or 13 percent of the population, are responsible for purchasing 70 percent of all over-the-counter medications, and they are very reluctant to tell us about the complementary therapies they may be taking. Much of the adverse effects and unusual problems can be related back to polypharmacy.

This subject is more complicated than just polypharmacy, however. In my ongoing review of the literature on this problem, I have not found one comprehensive study on adherence to medications with older cancer populations. We can extrapolate some from the general literature, but there is very little on this topic. When we think about what we give to our patients, medications for supportive care, for chemotherapy, biologics, analgesics, antiemetics, antibiotics, growth factors, chemoprotectants, psychoactives, and the impact all these drugs may have on functional decline, we should recognize the huge impact of altered pharmacokinetics and dynamics, drug misuse, nonadherence, and the prominence of adverse drug effects (Boyle, 2001). No one is coordinating all the medications that the older person is taking. I think this is an area particularly ripe for intervention.

Although the oral cancer drugs coming down the pipeline benefit older patients because they do not require visits for infusion, I worry that we also do not know if they take these medications. For example, in many medical oncology practices, I am told, when patients are given a prescription for their Xeloda (oral agent for metastatic breast cancer), they completely bypass the nurse for teaching; whereas, if they are prescribed an infusional drug, they see the nurse who explains when they have to come in, what to look for, and so on. So, somehow, there is this sense if it goes in your mouth it is maybe not as strong as when you get it in this tube going into a vein. So you do not have to worry about it, and, yet, when you look at the possibility of untoward effects with many of these drugs, it really is quite disconcerting.

To continue with the breast cancer example and adherence, so many decisions on the use of tamoxifen as an adjuvant treatment or for prevention of breast cancer are based on extensive clinical trial data. But how do we know those women took the agent as instructed? We really do not know; we just assume they did. There are so many possibilities for nonadherence: failure to fill the prescription, filling the prescription but not taking the medication, taking only a portion of the medication, failure to follow dose or frequency instructions, sharing the medication with someone with a similar health problem, substituting a former prescription, substituting an over-the-counter product, or deciding a prescription exceeds a personal preference on the number of prescriptions that are tolerable. There are also instances of misperception of instructions. One amusing one is the story of a man who was told to take all the pills in the bottle. When he returned for his next visit, he reported that he had done so, but that the last one was just too big to manage. It turned out that it was the preservative at the bottom of the bottle.

The implications of nonadherence to cancer treatment for outcomes were reviewed in 2002 (Partridge et al., 2002). For example, we could be attributing patient deterioration to lack of drug activity, when the problem may have been gaps in drug adherence. We see this in transplant patients. They stretch out the medication that is very expensive because they do not have the money to purchase it, even though Medicare may pay for 80 percent of it.

Lack of response to treatment may lead to unnecessary testing, dose changing, excess visits, and hospitalization. Hospital stays may be needlessly lengthened and misleading results obtained from clinical trials such as erroneous dosing recommendations or inconsistent response rates. There may be either increased toxicity due to over adherence—because more is always better—or decreased therapeutic efficacy or different kinds of compromised outcomes when patients are only partially adhering.

Symptom distress is the next issue. Exclusion of elderly people from clinical trials not only limits the evidence base on best treatments for our patients, but it also means we lack toxicity data, its prevalence, and optimal management. Also, comorbidities may confound symptom recognition. We see this in cancer survivors; we are uncertain whether a symptom is due to their comorbidity or whether it should be a concern that this new ache, pain, or symptom is due to a recurrence. Older patients may also be reluctant to report symptoms, since that implies that they are not doing well or are a complainer.

We also have problems with the tools that we use to measure symptom distress in the older population. We have some general gerontologic tools that are not sensitive or may not have been tested in the older cancer patient. We also have a comprehensive geriatric assessment that, in gerontology settings, takes 1.5 hours to complete. We will never get a busy medical oncologist to use something that complicated and time consuming. We need something more abbreviated and offering a significant return on the time and effort invested, perhaps something like the assessment that is being tested at Memorial or one that is being tested by advanced practice nurses in oncology across the United States. It is made up of Part I, which the patients complete before they come to clinic, and Part II, a validation that is done by the advanced practice nurse that covers medications, symptom distress, as well as functional status and many other measures we have heard about.

There is so much information on the geriatric syndromes in the general geriatric population that can be translated to the cancer population, and there is a whole realm of knowledge that we can be looking at related to the new issue of symptom clusters and intervention options based on how agents are metabolized.

Geriatric oncology and cancer survivorship share the feature that they are latecomers. The majority of people who survive cancer are elderly, and when we look at what kinds of cancers they had, a history of three primary solid tumors, breast, prostate, and colorectal, make up the majority. The older person's experience with survivorship is unstudied. This is where ageism comes in, despite the fact that they represent the largest number of survivors and will represent an even larger cohort in the future. We also know that by virtue of being old and having cancer, elderly people have a greater likelihood of developing a second or third primary tumor. And we know nothing about long-term effects of older patients who may go on to live another decade or two. We have no surveillance guidelines specific to some of the unique factors of the older patient.

Survivorship is a very nurse-intensive phenomenon because of the survivor's need for education, support, monitoring, integration of holistic approaches, and provision of care inclusive of the family. This was reviewed for the Institute of Medicine (IOM) in 2003 as part of the IOM's work on cancer survivorship (Ferrell et al., 2003).

And, lastly, there is end-of-life care. We may think older people think more about dying by virtue of seeing the hourglass run out, but that is not necessarily so. We know of many elderly who are very angry that they have cancer, and they expect to live another two decades. Frequently, the problem is that the children are not ready to let their mother go. So there is ambivalence about how their mother's treatment should be approached. Although we might like to think the majority of Americans benefit from hospice services, this is not true. More than half of all patients still continue to die in the acute care hospital, and we have not translated hospice care into a competency that is required of many of our inpatient staff.

I think ageism is involved here, too, when we look at the lack of assertiveness about confronting the quality of dying in older patients because we assume they are old and they are going to die. Let us focus our attention on someone who is younger. Looking at it very holistically, rather than just physiologically, often relief of terminal suffering is not achieved to the degree that it could be. I believe that the family's grief, particularly when the patient dies in the hospital, is directly linked with the circumstances of the patient's death. If it is not a good death, they are going to carry that memory with them for a long time. So I think we do not realize the power we have in helping to make the patient's death a good one in terms of both the patient and in terms of family bereavement and mourning. There are some interventions that we could use with our elderly patients that we historically have not used, such as reminiscence therapy.

In terms of building our capacity, we must have a partnership with gerontology. We need to make the community the focus of care, to test navigator roles by advanced practice nurses, to promote the integration of rehabilitation, to mandate a requirement in basic nursing programs, to engage in intensive partnerships with the family, and to develop and fund model programs.

Ageism can be confronted within the team when we hear it. Those kinds of biases and prejudices need to be confronted immediately. We can be measuring successes using nurse-sensitive outcomes such as management of symptoms, improvement of functional status, better patient safety, relief of psychological distress, and more efficient delivery of services. Recall that 55 percent of cancers now occur in 12 percent of Americans. Consider what that statistic will mean as the baby boomers begin to reach old age beginning in 2010, and the percent of elderly begins to increase to 20 or 30 percent. In the absence of any significant medical breakthrough, we can expect almost an epidemic of cancer, just by virtue of the changing demographics.

We need to be thinking about transition support, how we get patients into different settings with the support that is required. We also need to look at what I will call high-vulnerability risk profiles: patients that are being treated aggressively for leukemias and lymphomas with bone marrow transplantation. And we need to consider the community, the very high-risk cohorts that are old, female, poor, and African American, in terms of the many undue effects that happen to this population. We need to acknowledge and incorporate some of the advances that are possible with the sophisticated technical support that is in development.

In summary, those of us that work primarily with adult cancer patients do not think of ourselves as geriatric oncology nurses, but, in essence, we are. I believe that geriatric oncology nursing has come of age, and you will be seeing much more very innovative interventions from those of us in our specialty.

Dr. Ferrell: At the very beginning, you referred to a Geriatric Oncology Consortium. Could you say a little bit more about that because I was thinking we might want to share our report with them and get some feedback from them?

Ms. Boyle: It is an evolving group primarily made up of medical oncologists, and they actually are trying to develop the standard of care for older patients and improve on that standard with high-quality, age-sensitive clinical research. I am a member of their Scientific Advisory Board.

Currently, the majority of trials they have carried out have been in supportive care, looking at growth factor support as prophylaxis. Also, under Dr. Hyman Muss they have looked at first-line therapy for older women with metastatic breast cancer. The consortium is trying to generate interest in cancer in elderly people, and they have a counterpart in Europe, which is an international group with similar objectives.

Dr. Yancik: You mentioned Europe earlier, Deborah, in the context of talking about the instruments, and you said they are so far ahead of us. Perhaps I know what you are talking about with respect to the group. Would you like to say a little more about why you think they are so far ahead of us?

Ms. Boyle: The European Organization for Research and Treatment of Cancer (EORTC) has been devising and implementing elder-specific trials for perhaps two decades. Part of that, I think, has been generated by a partnership with geriatricians from the outset. Perhaps also because of their national health systems and the economics of limiting types of interventions, particularly chemotherapy, they have quite a long history of looking at elder-specific trials. And they have devised trials to look at some of the comorbidities and functional declines; so they are a great reference source. Several years ago, by comparison, I reviewed U.S. elderly cancer trials from the NCI cooperative groups and other sources such as the Pharmaceutical Research and Manufacturers of America (PhRMA). Admittedly, this may have improved somewhat since, but at the time I found seven such trials, quite a small number considering the numbers of elderly people.

Dr. Silliman: It may be worth mentioning to this group that the John A. Hartford Foundation, in collaboration with ASCO, funded eight programs around the country, including UCLA and Boston University (BU), to develop geriatric oncology training programs. So there are a few places around the country where people are being cross-trained. At BU, we graduate one fellow per year, so we are not going to make a huge dent very quickly in the workforce, but at least there is a small attempt to get people trained.

Dr. Barbara Given, Family Caregiving for Elderly Patients with Cancer: Existing Knowledge and Needed Research: I have organized what I want to talk about in two ways today. First, I want to tell you about our patients and their families and what they have told us over the last two decades, and, then, I want to raise the issues around research, intervention, and policy that I think need to be examined, given all the numbers we have seen today about what is going to happen in a few years.

In our work, I have defined family caregivers as those who provide uncompensated care in the home and who perform tasks of care, whether physical, emotional, social, or financial, for patients. In the United States, there are a few places that provide some compensation for individuals who provide care, but I am talking about those who are really uncompensated. And as has already been said, family members are involved in a wide variety of tasks and activities, sometimes 7 days a week, sometimes 24 hours a day. They are involved in 85 percent or more of cancer care. Even more important, perhaps, is the long duration of involvement in some circumstances, such as with dementia.

We do not think about cancer caregiving in terms of years, but if you examine caregiving from the initial diagnosis through therapy, potential progression, possible recurrence, and then perhaps even a second cancer or palliative care or end-of-life care, patients are involved with cancer a very long time. And when we have a second cancer or a late recurrence, family members tell us that they are already involved 4.6 years, on average. So, caregiving can go on for a considerable period of time, and as survivals lengthen to 15 or 20 years, as we have seen today, caregiving can stretch out for many years. So we have to think of the availability of family members. With smaller families and with the configurations that were mentioned this morning, the number of family caregivers who are going to be available in the future is going to be an issue.

The economic value of the family contribution in all situations, not just cancer, calculated at $9.92 per hour, was $306 billion in 2004 in that year's $1.878 trillion health expenditure. That is substantially more than what we are currently spending on nursing home care or home care. It is a major contribution and a major resource to the health-care system.

In thinking about the cancer care problem for elderly people, we need to remember that there are 6 million persons over age 65 alive with a history of cancer. Almost 840,000 individuals over 65 will be newly diagnosed with cancer in 2006, and almost 290,000 over 65 will die of the disease (69 percent of all cancer-related deaths). Comorbidities add complexity to this population of cancer patients, and some of them even have more than one cancer. All of these patients have affected family. So, we are talking about a great deal of care, many hours of care, and a significant contribution to our health-care system.

Factors affecting the family include the patients' physical health, and the fact that they have other chronic diseases, which adds to the comorbidity. We are all happy with the increased longevity, people living to be 80, 85, or 90, but this does add to the burden on caregivers. In our current study, we have family members and caregivers in their late 80s, and we have patients who are 91 who are cared for by adult daughters. As the health-care system moves to shortened hospital stays, we see more shifting of demand to families. Some patients may even complete their care without being hospitalized, and so the responsibility for care rests on family members. We have more complex home care, complex procedures, many ports and other complex devices. Oral agents can be taken at home, and that shifts care and adverse events back to the family and patients, and they may not know how to respond or how to differentiate between serious and minor complications.

There are community resources, but many of our community resources are not used by elderly people, even when they are available, because they are saving them for when they really need them. Or they may have experience with a previous chronic disease, and they recall that they were asked for a great deal of personal information, which now, as they read in the newspapers is the kind of thing that leads to identity theft, strangers coming into the home, or other worrisome possibilities. Furthermore, community resources are often not available in a way that is acceptable to them, either by how the calls are made or what happens during the very first visit. So they drop them, even when we believe that we have made them available.

Administration of a complicated regimen of oral agents would be complex for most of us, let alone a 70- or 80-year-old person who is taking up to 10 or 12 other medications. In addition, the out-of-pocket cost can be a real challenge. We heard earlier about nonadherence. We would probably all be shocked at what patients do, even with pain medications—the extent to which people do not take them for a variety of reasons, side effects, the confusion that occurs, or the cognitive effects of some of them.

I recently heard a story that illustrates some of these problems. An elderly woman had breast cancer surgery. She was prescribed codeine, but it caused her to be confused. She fell, broke her hip, and was admitted to a nursing home. She did not make progress in rehabilitation. So she was discharged. Now the major problem was no longer recovery from breast cancer surgery, but what the family could do about her fractured hip.

In sum, we find that family members and patients are less satisfied with their care. Much of the reason for that involves communication, either the lack of communication and understanding, not spending the time to communicate well, or nowadays under the Health Insurance Portability and Accountability Act (HIPAA) Privacy Rule, believing that certain family members—meaning the adult children—do not have the right to the data about their parent.

Care requirements bring about changes in the family; remember that in our work a third of all caregivers of elderly people are adult children, and they have other family and work roles to play, lives that they have to carry on. About a third of these caregivers report that they have a disturbance in their work due to emergency room visits, transportation of their parent, or other responsibilities that interfere with work. After the second or third round of this, it becomes a problem in the workplace. In our current study, we have a number of people who took care of their parent, did what was necessary, and then at the end found that their job was no longer there. We do not necessarily think about such things, but they can be critical, especially given the possibilities that co-payments and other out-of-pocket expenses can affect family finances and savings.

We think that people can automatically take on these roles and exercise the judgment that is required in providing care. But there are different judgments and different expectations of families in the acute phase, in the maintenance phase, in the rehab phase, the recurrence phase, or the palliative care phase at the end of life. There are different information requirements during these phases. So taking on one role and then knowing when to give up that role can be complicated. Knowing that the role is not to hover, and encouraging the patient to function more independently and not to be waited on is something that becomes a problem for family members. With each episode of care or each new diagnosis and each round of therapy, there may be new functional declines and disabilities that have to be faced.

What are the factors affecting caregiver distress? The research includes gender, relationship (adult children versus spouse), caregiver illness, and caregiver depression, and how these factors affect the care that is given or how caregivers report signs and symptoms or adverse events. The formal health-care system seldom becomes a partner with the family system or has a plan of care that includes family members. Most of the time, the geriatric assessment and plan of care do not include a family member role. Most of our intervention research has focused on reducing caregiver distress, when what we really need in our research are interventions that focus on how caregivers can affect outcomes by providing tailored care specific to the needs of the patient.

From other studies, we know that approximately one-third of the caregivers are quite burdened. We automatically assume there are more than that, because we hear a great deal from the burdened. A third of them are also clinically depressed. Many of them are not diagnosed, and they are not getting treated, even if depression is identified and is symptomatic at the level of clinical depression. An assessment question for the caregiver should be whether they currently are depressed or have been previously depressed, because depression affects the whole care trajectory. These studies show that caregiver distress can be at a very high level up to 18 months after care is completed. At that point, often another period of care is required, which renews the work role conflicts and other problems for the young adult children.

Among the factors that put family members at higher risk of inability to provide care over a long period of time is being a younger woman. They are more conflicted; they have competing roles; and they seem to have more depression, distress, and inadequate coping. Also included is being a nonspouse. The spouses and adult sons seem to do better. We also see fear of the future and worrying about death as factors, especially if the family has been having conflicts or impaired communication. In these situations, good relationships may get stronger, but it is unlikely that poor relationships will improve. Personality traits such as being naturally optimistic or pessimistic can be factors. Having resources and coming from a higher socioeconomic group can make a difference. If caregivers can buy support and assistance, they actually use more resources and can purchase respite to get them through times when they are stressed. Congruence between the perceived patient needs and the caregivers' perception of the patients' needs also varies, especially among the depressed caregivers. There have been several articles published recently showing as much as a 20 to 30 percent difference in how caregivers report symptoms. The more vague the symptom, the more discrepancy there is. Diarrhea or constipation are easy symptoms for them to agree on. Fatigue, depression, and others are more difficult for them to agree on.

Patient factors (we have talked about a number of these already today) that affect demand and caregiver distress include the amount of physical care required and changes in functional status. Some of the research shows that it is not so much the amount of physical care that is the issue; it is the constant transitions from more care to less care, less care to more care, or the number of changes that occur in a 12-month period.

The stage of disease is also important. Advanced stage disease is always more problematic for family members because of fears and uncertainty about what may happen. The number and severity of symptoms and the fact that pain and fatigue seem to drive number and severity, I think, dictate that, with some of our interventions, we need to target and work with family members on the management of pain and fatigue. Family caregivers tell us that they can deal with physical care and many other things, but depression and anger are two things that are difficult for them. Conflicts and inconsistency on decisions among providers are emotionally wearing too.

We do not think about disruptive behavior in cancer patients. That is more in dementia. But, there are brain tumors with cognitive effects, and certainly the delirium that comes with some of the medications and polypharmacy can be disruptive. These things are problems for family members of cancer patients. We have talked about geriatric syndromes such as falls, incontinence, and delirium, and I gave the example of the hip fracture. And we have talked about comorbidity.

In addition to caregiver factors and patient factors affecting caregiver distress and the care that is delivered, there are the specifics of the care situation that can have an impact on caregiver distress and performance. These include the hours of care or the vigilance that is required and how many hours during the day vigilance is required to ensure adherence to medications, required physical activity, or other rehabilitation or treatment programs. Often there is no respite. For the older spouses, there is the feeling that they cannot turn over the care to someone else or they will feel guilty if they do because it is their role and responsibility to take care of their spouse. They are afraid to go to church. They are afraid to go out because something might happen. We have already mentioned the formal health-care system. Often the formal home care referrals reviewed in our medical record audits are not consistent with patient need at discharge or later. Social support can also be lacking.

As discussed earlier, the physical care required is often not the most difficult burden for family members to deal with. We ask family members to provide types of care that, for those of us who are nurses, we would not let our beginning nursing students do without supervision. Yet, we often send family members home with very little guidance, counseling, or direction about what to do, and we do not give them the range of expectations. How many diarrhea stools are too many? How many skin lesions are too many? Fever of how high? And as a result they have so much anxiety about knowing what to do and fearing that they are going to use the system too much.

There is such a broad range of things that we are expecting them to be responsible for because they are only coming in every 3 to 6 weeks on their protocols, and in between times, it is up to them. If they need guidance, they get in a queue on the answering system, and they may be hours waiting, may not be called back the same day, or may be called back, not by their own nurse who has their record in front of her, but by the phone nurse who has a protocol that we designed to deal with the symptom, not the individual who is actually there.

Some of the direct care activities that they are responsible for, varying in the amount of time they take and the judgment that they require, include: medication dispensing and monitoring; symptom management and monitoring of side effects and adverse events; meal preparation and nutritional balance; care decisions and problem solving; skin care and infection control; management of highly technical equipment and medical procedures such as catheters and wound care; bill paying; and transportation and errands.

We have many documents these days on patient safety and quality of care. We think about those issues in the formal health-care system. But, as we consider what we expect of the patient and the family, we should remember they are not in the formal system. I can not find studies on quality indicators for family members or studies that have even gauged the quality of care from family members. We need to begin looking at, or at least projecting, which situations may support good quality of care and good patient safety and in which situations we may need to be cautious or we believe there are high-risk factors for negative outcomes. Caregivers need some knowledge for symptom management, accessing the health-care system appropriately, and coordination of care. They need to know about prevention and early detection of complications and adverse events, among other things.

We have many studies on caregiver stress, burden, adjustment, and coping. We have many breast cancer studies. We have a fair number of prostate cancer caregiving studies. We have very few lung cancer studies, and we probably have more palliative care studies. But we need to look at some of the other conditions. I think the needs of our many brain cancer patients warrant examination. We have virtually no studies that explore interventions that are trying to improve skills for care and family problem solving, and we do not have many studies that really look at facilitating movement across the transition phases of care. Most of the intervention studies for caregivers are anticipatory guidance and education.

We know that the most effective intervention studies in dementia, for example, are multimodal studies of a variety of strategies, with education, cognitive, behavioral, and problem solving included. We need those in cancer as well as dementia; I think we can learn from the dementia work that has been done for elderly people. We know who is at risk for the burden of cancer caregiving, and we know some of who gives the care and what care is given, although we have not formally looked at the tasks of care and the percentage of time spent in the various tasks of care across the stages of cancer. Not all care is problematic. We have a few studies that indicate that you can be burdened, but yet receive some rewards out of the value of caring and the feeling of a positive contribution. Not all caregivers are distressed, and I think it would be worthwhile to look at those who are not distressed and figure out why. Who are they? What are the characteristics that allow them to get through some very horrendous situations and still stay on top of it and avoid distress?

The intervention studies today have very few good descriptions. It is very difficult to enroll and retain distressed caregivers. As was mentioned earlier, the distressed patients or the patients who are not doing well drop out of studies. We need to figure out how we get to the people most in need. We need to know what interventions work and what the dosing, titration, or tailoring of those interventions should be. You will not find any caregiving studies that describe the intervention in enough detail to really know those things. I could find no caregiving studies in cancer that looked at patient outcomes as a result of that care, with one possible exception.

We need to look at how caregiver skills change across diagnosis. We need to look at patient outcomes as well as the caregiver outcomes, because the system is going to care about the patient outcomes first, since that is where the payment is. I think CMS should collect information on these performance measures too. But then we would need standards and guidelines for family care and the quality of family care. I think ASCO and the National Comprehensive Cancer Network (NCCN) should work on those. We have examined the cost of few caregiver interventions, and there have been few formal home health-care studies. These could be worthwhile. For care situations that are not working, where the family members are overusing the health-care system as a check on their performance or for respite, it would be valuable to know the cost and compare that cost with the potential cost of educational or guidance programs that would help to prevent such expensive behavior. We have, in our studies, certain family members that use the emergency room as a security blanket every time something happens, rather than problem solve. There are few formal home care studies that examine cancer patients. Many involve congestive heart failure or COPD, but few look at cancer.

With regard to methodological limitations, most studies cover a variety of diagnoses and stages. So you might find an intervention study on people who are diagnosed 6 months to 17 years ago. We find very little impact in most of those intervention studies, but there has not been any deconstruction of the interventions. So, in these studies that do not have wonderful outcomes, we need to look at subgroups and subsamples.

We have few longitudinal studies. It is expensive to follow patients and family members across transitions, but I think we need to do that, and I think we need to have studies that link the caregiver interventions with patients' clinical outcomes and look at the value added. Our future research needs to look specifically at some of the patient outcomes, such as symptoms, function, cost utilization, and complications, and measure the quality of those. We need to examine which of the expected outcomes for patients are sensitive to family members' care. When does family members' care make a difference? I would recommend that we consider family member care as a supportive care agent for patients' clinical outcomes.

In addition, we need to look at ethnic and cultural variations and disparities. There are very few of those studies that have been carried out, and fewer yet with patients or family members in disparity situations. In Michigan, few of those patients come to the cancer centers, and so there is difficulty in reaching them. We think that some of the people with disparities are costing the system a great deal, and I can assure you they are not getting the care they need.

I think we need to examine the skill levels of family members and how that affects outcomes. Not all family members and not all aged caregivers have the requisite skills. For example, we have in our church a woman treated for breast cancer, and her husband needs to go on hospice for prostate cancer. This has resulted in a controversy as to whether he can use hospice because his wife is not going to be available enough to provide the care. What happens if caregivers have negative reactions? Can they get involved in care? We have looked at clinically depressed patients and caregivers. The congruence between the reporting of the symptoms is way off, and the patient outcome and symptom severity at the end of our nursing intervention was far worse than those where one or the other of the two dyads was not depressed. And, then, I would like to see some studies where we really try a partnership between the formal system and the informal system in the care plan.

I think we need to look at the different skills that are required across the trajectory. As I said earlier, one set of skills does not fit for every stage of disease, nor for every patient, nor for every diagnosis. We need to look at which interventions work best in which situations. When does problem solving work best? When does social support work best? When does counseling work best? And when does a combination of those things work best? Taking those things into consideration, we need to prescribe interventions as we do drugs. We need to look at when is the best time for caregiver interventions. When they are depressed or distressed? Before? How soon? How early, and when do you get the best look? Timing has not been in our intervention research.

The effect on caregivers' health has not been examined in cancer at all and has been done little in dementia. How many cancer caregivers are taking psychotropic agents as a quick fix? We see distressed caregivers using their primary doctors more, but they are not being evaluated in their caregiving role. They are being treated for whatever else is manifested by stress, such as GI symptoms or headaches. We have not seen so much prescribing of psychotropics or hypnotics. What about inattention to their own chronic diseases—the diabetic who is in or out of control, the hypertensive who is in or out of control, and putting off their own cancer screening? We need to look at opportunity costs to families through multiple-year care roles. My example is the adult daughter who was in line for a principalship in the Lansing school system. When she got there, her mother was diagnosed with ovarian cancer, and she gave up her principalship. Of course, her mother soon died, and she was very angry because she thought we should have told her, and maybe we did and she did not hear it. Anyway, she never got back in line in that school system again. She had passed up her opportunity. And then the people who, in our current study, have lost their jobs: what will happen to them? Who has the health insurance affects decisions that family members make for promotions, for moves, and for other important things when there is a diagnosis of cancer. Those are influences that should not be treated lightly.

Future research should look at the response by a spouse or adult child to late effects when the survivor is an 80-year-old whose first cancer might have been at age 60 or 65. I have not talked much at all about how technology (electronic) aids can assist caregivers (reducing anxiety and depression) and lead to better outcomes. In dementia and some of the other chronic diseases, there are many good websites and many good support groups for family caregivers. The NCI recently issued a couple of booklets specific to family caregiving in cancer, but I do not think we have enough interventions with technology aids and assistance to think about in relation to outcomes. I mentioned earlier, decision making and quality of care with distressed compared to nondistressed caregivers. What choice of outcome should we look at for the family caregiver? We have focused on burden, distress, and depression. Should it be capacity, maybe? What other kinds of things could we look at, and what could be outcomes?

We need to think about variation in skills, because what works when a person is requiring a great deal of emotional support from a family member is different than when they are at end of life or in palliative care. Sometimes, adult children are not as good at certain phases as spouses or other caregivers. We sometimes see sons and daughters who do not like the phase of physical care, and they need assistance. We need to know, to classify, the knowledge and skills that family members need, maybe by diagnosis, certainly by stage, and then figure out ways both for research and also how best to reach the caregivers who are overwhelmed. Finally, we need to remember that family members are an excellent resource. Although we may not acknowledge it, they are a hidden resource for the health-care system, a part of our care.

Dr. Cruz: It sounds wonderful. Who is going to pay for changing the system to do this? Even to do the studies is a challenge given the state of NCI funding.

Dr. Given: I doubt anyone is going to pay for this in my lifetime, but I do believe that it might be possible to build inexpensive ways into our current system if we can systematize what may work; technology may be important to think about. In England, they give family members a personal digital assistant (PDA) for management of a patient's symptoms when they think the patient is going to have difficulty, and what comes up, then, on the PDA are some strategies to help manage pain or whatever the symptom is.

Dr. Ganz: I think one of the problems is the fragmentation of our health-care system: different payors paying, or not paying, for different services related to informal caregiving. Have you thought about working within an integrated health-care delivery system where the payoff for keeping services in the family rather than delivering them in the emergency room or some other part of the formal system could be measured? I am thinking of the Henry Ford or Kaiser system, for example, because I think those systems might be motivated to test some of these interventions where they can account for the savings.

Dr. Given: We have not been to Henry Ford or Kaiser, but we approached the Blue Cross Insurance plans in Michigan, and they said they did not have enough cancer patients in any one location, and the difficulty of their systems communicating with one another would make it difficult to gather information on time, place, and cost of various services.

Dr. Robinson: These issues transcend cancer. They show up in Alzheimer's patients and many other patients with serious chronic conditions. It seems, because it is such a widespread problem, that there should be some way of aligning the interests of others with similar concerns to begin to define possible solutions.

Dr. Kathleen Foley: End of Life Care: End-of-life care in the cancer patient is an example of a generic issue that, I believe, provides a model to improve the health-care system by focusing on the cancer population and learning and demonstrating better patterns of care. So it is an opportunity. When I was on the National Cancer Policy Board, we wrote a report called

Improving Palliative Care for Cancer, and we made a number of recommendations. Some of these were accepted, but they all need to be, because they are critically important. There is, as well, an IOM study, *Approaching Death: Improving Care at the End of Life,* that examines palliative care as a generic issue across all diseases, including cancers, and serves as a model with a set of recommendations, which also have been addressed only in part. And, lastly, there are some really terrific books out there. One by Joanne Lynn, *Sick to Death and Not Going to Take It Anymore: Reforming Health Care in the Last Years of Life,* is a practical book about the need to change the health-care system to focus on this.

While end-of-life care is a health-care system issue, the cancer establishment should not give up on it. It is about quality cancer care, and one of our problems is that for those who are not candidates for surgery or chemotherapy there is no quality cancer care, and, particularly not at the end of life, and it seems to me that we could do better.

So here is the example of an 88-year-old man living in an assisted-living center with his 86-year-old wife with dementia. He was in relatively good health and was cognitively intact. She has a massive left hemisphere stroke and is transferred to a hospital and then discharged to a nursing home. He is left in the assisted living. He, then, develops progressive back pain, fatigue, and anorexia and is diagnosed with pancreatic cancer that prevents him from staying in this assisted-living center. The center, which wants nothing to do with him at this point, strongly advises that he be transferred to the nursing home where his wife is. But the nursing home, then, is profoundly challenged by managing his symptoms, as are his primary care physicians, because they have got an elderly patient with pancreatic cancer, and they are not sure how to take care of this patient. And that is where the system falls apart. I think the cancer establishment should address this kind of thing if we want to improve cancer care.

I will give you a second example of the craziness of the system. This is a 90-year-old woman cared for in a hospice program with cancer and a prognosis of less than six months. She went on to live for three years, but was followed by the hospice program. The hospice program was investigated by the government and accused of fraud because they were continuing to provide hospice care for someone with a fatal diagnosis who did not die. This was a small hospice program and the only one in a relatively rural city in upstate New York, and the government stopped providing funding to this program. Only after the *Wall Street Journal* reported this on its front page was there congressional outrage and some change.

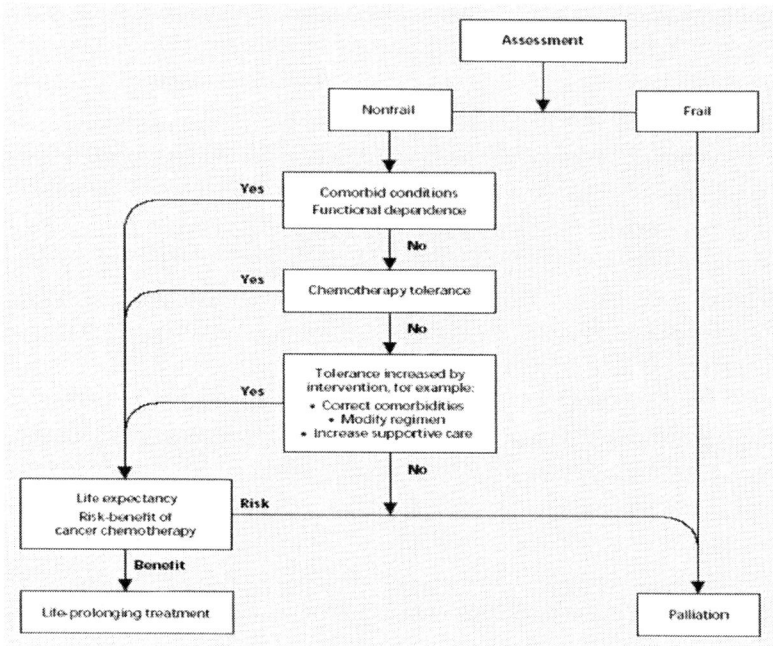

FIGURE 2-12 Algorithm for managing older patients with cancer.
SOURCE: Foley, 2006; from Balducci, 2003.

Figure 2-12 is an example of one algorithm for managing older patients with cancer. Unfortunately, the initial construct separates patients into frail or nonfrail. The frail will get palliation, but there is no definition of this palliation in any detail, and the nonfrail will go through a series of decisions and may or may not get treatment without defining very clearly what we mean by life-prolonging treatment versus palliation.

The models for geriatric cancer care need to be made more sophisticated. I support using a comprehensive geriatric assessment. The assessments that are currently being used include functional status, comorbidity, socioeconomic issues, nutritional status, polypharmacy, and geriatric syndromes. However, they need also to consider a good symptom assessment scale, information about the patient's shared decision-making process, where patients stand on advance directives, and goals of care. This is an opportunity where palliative care and geriatrics can come together, although, the National Institute on Aging repeatedly tells me that they focus on aging, and dying is not something they want to talk about.

How do we interface geriatrics and palliation? I think the domains clearly involve access to care, patient-centered care, and some ethical issues that are at the forefront and need a great deal of discussion and leadership: issues of nutrition and hydration, of sedation, where physician-assisted suicide and euthanasia really come to the fore. They are part of the public fabric of our discussions about these issues—involving the role of volunteers, funding, research, and challenges to organizational structures. Clearly, some open, transparent discussions about these are critically important.

Figure 2-13 displays the formalized, integrated model that addresses both curative and palliative care for chronic progressive illness. In the care of the cancer patient we should build into the algorithm in Figure 2-12 that patients, depending on their needs, will receive palliative care. This is different than supportive care, which, in the cancer literature, is about treating symptoms caused by chemotherapy; it is about blood products. There should be explicit data about the use of supportive therapies, but they are not palliative care services. There are clear national guidelines for palliative

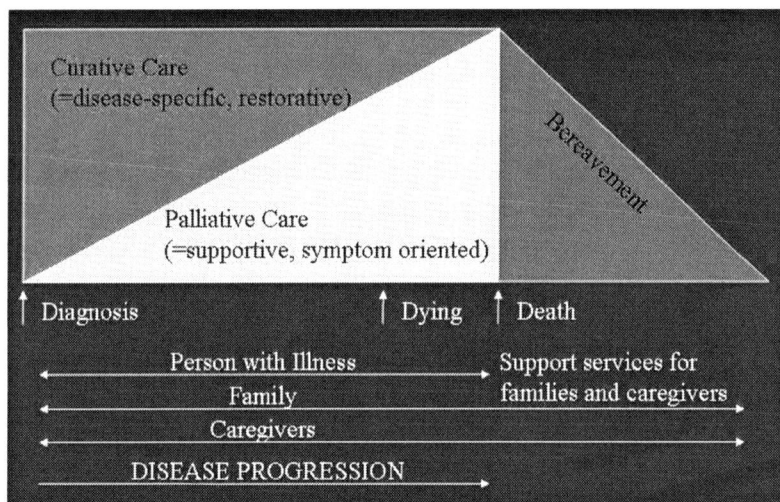

FIGURE 2-13 Integrated model for chronic progressive illness.
SOURCE: WHO Expert Committee, 1990.

care and guidelines for who should receive that care. These need to be interfaced more closely with geriatrics.

The opportunity is to take the lead and provide end-of-life care for the cancer patient that can be a model for other chronic illnesses and to do it by dealing with patients over time in a trajectory of care. Models are now developing in what is called simultaneous care. Patients who could be candidates for a phase 1 trial can simultaneously receive palliative care therapies and then transfer into hospice at some appropriate time in relation to the trial. Evidence suggests that this is very cost-effective and limits the amount of time such patients might require inpatient hospitalization. This argument is not simply an economic one, it is also about quality of care.

Much is happening at an international level that has focused on elderly people. The World Health Organization (WHO) in Europe has argued strongly for palliative care within the cancer population, as well as the geriatric population, and very specifically for better palliative care for older people, emphasizing the critically important aspects for the cancer population. They are moving forward on guidelines that focus on palliative care for elderly people and defining what that should look like, making palliative care a public health priority and building it into national cancer control strategies. The foundation for all this involves challenges for public policy makers and the broader constructs of the rights and the needs of older people, issues of underassessment and treatment, and evidence for effective care solutions. In Norway, the United Kingdom, and Sweden, for example, I think there are better models, including economic models that we might look into.

The British have a proportionately larger population of older people than the United States, and 75 percent of cancer deaths occur in the over 65 population.

In the United States, the SEER data do not tell us the patients' place of death, how long they were there, or the quality of care. But the British do have some data, and what they are seeing over time in the older cancer patients is an increasing return to hospital for treatment and for care at the end-of-life (close to 50 percent of deaths at ages 65–94 in 1999) in spite of ready access to hospice or end-of-life units in hospitals. They are enormously concerned about this, and it has to do with the therapies that are now being offered and the toxicity of those therapies that requires return to care.

One of the issues that we have to balance is that, in providing such treatment and recognizing that, for the most part, cancer care in the United

States has become an outpatient service, elderly people cannot stay at home. Home health services do not work. They cannot get hospice care because they are getting active therapy, and the hospital is the only place they can go. We are, in effect, creating a movement back to hospital deaths, with the enormous costs that go with that, and we need to look at that cost shifting.

The European Federation of Older Persons is playing a major role in defining a palliative care program. The distinction between the European system and the American system is critical. In the European systems—Sweden, Norway, and Britain—or more widely in the world, for example, in Australia and Canada—concurrent hospice and palliative care and active cancer treatment are possible. Concurrent hospice and active treatment is not available in the United States, and that is why the European model is useful, because they have some economic data that might help us move forward.

The Hastings Center published a report, *Improving End-of-Life Care: Why Has It Been So Difficult?* Death is always a second choice for Americans who want liberty first ("Give me liberty or give me death"), but I think we could be smarter about it. The movement for formal advance directives would be an approach. According to data from the Brown Medical School website (http://www.chcr.brown.edu/dying/MAPADALL.htm) examining formal advance directives in populations in nursing homes (which are, with hospitals, one of the two most common sites of death for cancer patients over age 75), there is incredible variation across the country.

This variation is due to difficulties in advance care planning and depends significantly on variable state laws but also on difficulties in communication between physicians and patients regarding goals and likely outcomes, contingency plans, and the specifics of patient age and condition. This process has become a complicated, cultural, medical process that has to happen, and so the movement afoot is to do it within this framework that requires greater sophistication in cancer. I think cancer leaders should take this on with the cancer population. The public needs an engagement in communication and better negotiation about goals and likely outcomes.

My advocacy is for the older patient to have the options that anyone would have, that we do not discriminate because of age, that they would have the option for every therapy and participation in clinical trials. This requires communication and a negotiation about goals, specifying targets to patients' age and their conditions, recognizing their significant limitations, and understanding it is not a single conversation and that there need to be contingency plans. This is the new framework that is attempting to structure advance planning better. About 45 percent of cancer patients have advance directives. This is much higher than the general population, so they have already made progress. What do we have to do to get to 70 percent or 80 percent and to review the usefulness of this process?

Communication and negotiation—where am I in my disease course? Have I reached a critical turning point? What are the goals of care? Has a contingency plan been formulated to honor the patient's preferences? All of this has to be done in the setting of family decision making. The data suggest this is all about family decision making, not even patient decision making.

What about research support for palliative care? There have been two state-of-the-science meetings, one in 2002 and one in 2004 (http://consensus.nih.gov/PREVIOUSSTATEMENTS.htm). A study supported by the U.S. Cancer Pain-Relief Group looked at NIH funding and reported that less than one percent of NIH funding (most of it in the NCI) goes to pain or symptom management. This number has not changed, no matter what recommendations we have made.

When research or career development funding for geriatrics is compared with funding for palliative care, the huge majority is for geriatrics. Perhaps we could balance this a bit more and devote somewhat more to research and career development in palliative care. Legislation has been introduced in Congress called the Palliative Care Training Act. This act would create hospice and palliative care academic career awards. We should encourage the development of these career development awards to begin to move this forward. I am making this distinction because there is much overlapping. If you compare the field of geriatrics and its principles and the

TABLE 2-7 Odds of Surviving 2 Months After Prognoses from 1 to 7 Days

Days Before Death	Median Patient's Odds of Surviving 2 Months
1	1:8
2	1:4
3	1:3
7	1:2

SOURCE: Adapted from Foley, 2006; adapted from SUPPORT Principal Investigators, 1995.

field of palliative care, they are closely aligned. So we should not see such a discrepancy in these kinds of funding strategies, and we should think about a way to improve them.

Why is this so difficult? We are not very skilled at determining when someone will die. Table 2-7 shows the odds of surviving an additional two months after prognoses of 1-, 2-, 3-, or 7-days. Given a 7-day prognosis, patients have a 50 percent chance of living another 2 months. This exemplifies the problem we have of predicting who is dying. We have to create a system that is not dependent upon how soon someone is going to die, but at the moment we have a Medicare hospice benefit that is still predicated on a 6-month life span. Joanne Lynn and others have argued for a policy called Medicaring that focuses on burden of disease and functional disability, not on timing. I think that is a wise statement of policy, although the current Medicare hospice benefit is what we have, and it works well for many patients. We do not want to damage what we have. But we could make it better, and cancer seems like the disease to demonstrate improvements and perhaps save money in the process.

How is cancer different? In cancer, a period of stability is followed by functional decline and death. Cancer patients experience a relatively constant declining trajectory to death. This compares with a fluctuating declining and recovering and declining course of congestive heart failure. With this kind of information, we probably could create prediction models for cancer. For example, we have data to show that activities of daily living also are stable and then decline rapidly as death approaches for cancer patients compared to congestive heart failure, stroke, COPD, or diabetes. Similarly, cancer patients after a period of stability decline rapidly in their ability to get in and out of bed or a chair compared to that same group of conditions.

The same is true for dependent activities of living. In a study of a cohort of established populations older than 65 years (Lunney et al., 2003), those with sudden death maintained good function throughout the last year of life; those with organ failure had fluctuating declines with a deterioration in the last three months; frail decedents were relatively more disabled in the final year, and cancer patients were highly functional during the first part of the last year, but sustained marked declines in the last three months. Cancer patients and the frail elderly appear somewhat similar, but the cancer patients tail off more rapidly. I am making the argument that cancer is a little bit different, because you can prognosticate, and it has a rather sharp decline. It gives you, then, an opportunity to study it as different from other diseases.

There is another way cancer is different. Symptoms such as pain, dyspnea, nausea, and vomiting are much more prevalent in the last week of life of cancer patients. In general populations of patients that are older versus those with a specific cancer diagnosis, symptoms such as cognitive impairment, loss of bladder and bowel control, visual and auditory symptoms, and dizziness are more prevalent.

Symptoms reported most often among people in residential homes at some point in their last year of life include mental confusion, constipation, dribbling, bad temper, and difficulty hearing or seeing. These data suggest that symptom management research could be focused on the specifics of different age populations and what they need most.

Pain has been quite problematic in the elderly population. About 41.2 percent of nursing home residents who have pain on their first assessment experience moderate daily pain or excruciating pain on their second assessment. This is persistent pain in cancer patients in nursing homes, and statistics on pain in nursing home patients vary considerably across the United States. So we have very cancer-specific data; therefore, we have the opportunity to perform interventions that would be very specific to the cancer population.

We also have discovered that if you put a hospice in a skilled nursing facility, the hospice residents are 70 percent less likely to be hospitalized. There have been discussions about end-of-life care. There have been goals of care set, and those patients are getting care to their wishes and needs. They are twice as likely to have pain assessed and treated, and they experience significantly fewer intrusive medical interventions. Hospice residents scored significantly higher than nonhospice residents on all symptom management outcomes. So there is much greater attention to the goals of care for the individual patients if a hospice program is available. Clearly, a hospice care system can provide patients with appropriate quality care that is critically necessary.

What happens in this elderly population with cancer? They typically are initially cared for at home. Then they are admitted to hospital. Then they go to a skilled nursing facility, and they may end up at home, in hospice care, or in a nursing home. When bereaved family members were interviewed regarding their perception about the level and pattern of distressing pain at the last two sites of care, 40 percent were reported to have had distressing pain in the last site, and about 42 percent had it at their second site. The evidence is consistent regarding inadequate pain management, and apparently a change to another place of care does not result in improved management.

Why is this? There are multiple reasons, but pain syndromes are due both to their incurable chronic conditions and to their cancer. The difficulty of prescribing analgesics in patients with cognitive impairment and metabolic and pharmacodynamic changes is considerable, and we do not have guidelines for opioids in elderly people. It is very difficult to receive funding for studies of opioids in elderly people. Cognitive dysfunction clearly complicates symptom assessment, although there are models now for pain assessment in the cognitively impaired, and psychosocial issues such as depression are significant both in the caregivers as well as in the patients.

There are good data, the minimum datasets in nursing homes, that allow patients with cancer to be identified. The residents with cancer are about 80, the same age as the residents without cancer. The cancer patients are more than twice as likely (45 percent versus 17 percent) as the national average to have advance directives, suggesting that they have been more thoughtful and focused on these issues. Only about four percent in the nursing home are receiving chemotherapy, but a higher percent are getting some type of intravenous medication. They are requiring oxygen and nutrition, and some are on feeding tubes. These are all care decisions that need to be addressed as to whether they are appropriate. Is it what the patients and families wanted and what has resulted from good communication? Pain in this population is clearly the dominant symptom.

So, we have data that should allow us to develop guidelines for appropriate quality care of seriously ill and dying patients to provide the desired level of physical comfort and emotional support, to support shared decision making, to treat the individual with respect, to provide emotional support to the family, and to coordinate care across settings. And so these are, in a way, outcome measures that one could use to begin to assess care. In fact, an attempt has been made to do this in a large dataset in which caregivers were questioned about family perspectives on care at the last place of care. Family members responsible for 67 percent of the patients reported that their patient was in an institution as the last site of care. Although, the intent of hospice is to allow patients to die at home, the reality is that elderly people are dying in institutions, be it a hospital or a nursing home. Twenty-five percent were reported by family members to have had pain or dyspnea inadequately treated, and 33 percent of the family members had inadequate emotional support. Family members reported better satisfaction with the quality of care for hospice compared to either institutional care or home health care. If they were able to receive hospice care in a nursing home or in a home situation, they preferred that.

How families make difficult decisions about hospice enrollment and what patients and families want to know have been studied (Casarett et al., 2005). The majority of patients over age 65 (48 percent of whom were cancer patients) and their families had no knowledge of hospice at the time of the initial hospice visit. So as much as we think that we have penetrated the country with knowledge about hospice care, this study tells us how little is known.

The degree to which decisions were shared varies widely. Family members play a major role, and patients and families have very predictable patterns of informational needs. In this study, patients who had serious illness were given information about hospice care independent of their physicians and of the system in which they were. With this simple intervention, 20 percent of the residents were moved into hospice within a 30-day period versus 3 percent of those who were not so informed, and they spent less time in the acute care setting and benefited more the earlier the referral. An intervention that was purely educational allowed for a greater acceptance of hospice care, which indicates that there is undereducation of the populace and underadvocacy for this approach. The IOM report on palliative care identified physicians as one of the major problems in this respect.

What do families want to know? They want to know how often, if the patient is at home, will he or she receive a home visit? Who is going to pay? What kind of practical help is available to patients and families? What is the continuity of treatment? In the end, 67 percent of the decisions were made, or mostly made, by the family rather than the patient. Only about 23 percent were made, or mostly made, by the patient. The remaining 11 percent of the decisions were shared equally. Is this pattern of decision making because of cognitive impairment or some other problem in the individual patient? How do we help facilitate a shared decision making approach? Because the plurality of the decisions were made in a hospital (45 percent), we need to know how developed the approaches are at the hospital for explaining the choices and how they can be implemented. Nevertheless, I am encouraged that we are beginning to discuss and study some of these issues.

In England, a 27-item survey of preferences in end-of-life care has been developed to interview older patients as a method to begin to address what patients would want, as opposed to just families. Patients surveyed in this way seemed to be relatively knowledgeable about hospice care. They did not want doctors to assist the dying process, however. These views do not seem to explain underutilization of hospice (Catt et al., 2005).

Another questionnaire assessed the differences between African Americans over the age of 65 years and Caucasians with metastatic cancer in attitudes toward end-of-life care and survival, what kind of care and what kind of decision making they wanted, and what they wanted from their physicians (Hwang et al., 2003). African Americans were less likely to complete advance directives, to have knowledge about hospice, and to feel capable of assessing their health situation. There clearly are disparities in the access to hospice care, knowledge about hospice care, and the decision making about these issues for the African American population, where it has been best studied, and some data suggest similarities in the Hispanic population.

As for a research agenda, Goldstein and Morrison, noting that the evidence base for palliative care in older people is sparse, suggested major areas that should be addressed, including establishing the prevalence of symptoms in patients with chronic disease; evaluating the association between treatment of symptoms and outcomes; increasing the evidence base for treatment of symptoms; understanding psychological well-being, spiritual well-being, and quality of life of patients, elucidating and alleviating sources of caregiver burden; reevaluating service delivery; adapting research methodologies specifically for geriatric palliative care; and increasing the number of geriatricians trained as investigators in palliative care research (Goldstein and Morrison, 2005).

So I will conclude by saying that I think there is an opportunity to use the cancer population, for which we have a great deal of data, as a model of how we can improve the system of care. We have sufficient evidence to argue for that, and there is a beginning with the CMS discussions and demonstration projects as well as some international models.

Dr. Ferrell: This month, the National Quality Forum Guidelines on Palliative Care will be released. The forum basically took the National Consensus Project Clinical Practice Guidelines for Palliative Care the next step forward and created preferred practices that could lead to specific, measurable outcomes. I am interested in moving this discussion forward, not just by laying out issues, but to say what could be done. From what has been said today, it seems that we can conclude collectively that older people with cancer, even those who have the best prognosis and may become long-term cancer survivors, need the combination of palliative care with the best of cancer care. Applying the preferred practices from the National Quality Forum to geriatrics and older people with cancer as a demonstration and a challenge to our cancer centers would be one good way to do that.

Let us build on something that has just happened. The preferred practices have been through extensive peer review. Now, there are a number of efforts moving forward to ensure that we have outcome measures to measure the preferred practices. I think implementation of the practices would be an important thing to pursue following this meeting.

Dr. Foley: I totally agree, but in my mind, they are not enough.

Dr. Ferrell: Yes, they are not the only steps, but we should give people a template, a road map of preferred practices that would improve clinical care. I agree that we still need the research piece and other things that have been discussed today.

Dr. Benz: When you talk about nursing homes, are you talking just about skilled nursing facilities or about assisted-living facilities and other places? There is a growing population that presents for cancer care that in certain ways is the worst of all possible worlds because the home caregiver still has much of the burden. There is not a great deal of skilled care available, but some of the issues of being institutionalized also apply to them.

Dr. Foley: There are no good studies available on assisted living and cancer care. In a way, that is the growth market. It seems to me that every assisted-living corporation in the country wants to retain cancer expertise to create support for residents. I think that is a business model moving forward.

What I am talking about is research. We do not have minimum datasets from assisted-living facilities as we do from nursing homes, which are regulated in an intensive and different way. This, unfortunately results in their not wanting any patient to die in their institution, or, if they do die, only after interventions that prolong the process because they are so reluctant to have any deaths in the first place. I think the regulations that control the nursing homes interfere with good care of cancer patients. That is the problem.

There is no regulation of assisted-living facilities at the present time, except for the work of nurses and health-care delivery that occurs there and is regulated in a different way. I think business people are looking into clever assisted-living models of how a cancer chemotherapy nurse or any one of a variety of similar things could be provided.

Dr. Yates: Thirty years ago, in Vermont, we showed in a comparative trial that you could get two-thirds of the patients dying at home if you provided proper home support, compared to one-third in a control group. The biggest single question was what to expect. As long as there was interaction with the nurses, and the family felt comfortable that they were not going to be suddenly faced with a last-minute crisis, they were okay.

My second comment is that the 6-month limit on hospice imposed by the (then) Health Care Financing Administration (HCFA) was a reaction to a concern about overuse by home health agencies, because the one advantage of hospice over customary care is sending nurses into the home to provide support. The experience in the 1960s was that home health agencies used this to bill for excessive services, and so the limitation was a reaction to that.

Dr. Ya-Chen Tina Shih, Associate Professor of Biostatistics, MD Anderson Cancer Center: Economics of Cancer in the Elderly Population: What do I mean by the economics of cancer? Most economists have quantitative training to deal with how to allocate limited resources efficiently and equitably. Interestingly, efficiency and equity do not always go together; often there is a trade-off involved in those economic decisions. Many of the studies looking at the economics of cancer focus on cost-effectiveness analysis (CEA). Some look at the profitability of oncology practice.

I want to point out today that economic studies are much more than just CEAs. For example, economists care about how financial incentives change the behavior of patients or of providers, thus triggering a different treatment pattern. Economists also care about disparities in the financial burdens for different cancer families. They also care about the economics of the oncology workforce. The ultimate goal of economic study is to come up with policy recommendations through rigorous analysis of available evidence.

Today, I will review the literature on the following four areas: the economic burden of cancer; the economics of cancer prevention in the elderly population; the economics of cancer treatment in the elderly population;

and I will end with very brief comments on supply-side considerations. In reviewing the literature, I want also to consider the following four factors that might have an impact on what we observe or can expect to observe in the future. These are the technology factors, including the many technology advances and treatment pattern variations in cancer; the biological factors, especially to be considered in elderly people, such as coexisting medical conditions and physiological changes of aging; the policy factors such as the Medicare Modernization Act and the Medicare Prescription Drug Plan (also known as Part D), that will have an important impact on our healthcare system; and the factor of increasing diversity in our population, which raises concerns about disparities.

Every year, the NCI reports the total cost of cancer in three categories. One is the direct medical cost. These are costs related to prevention, diagnosis, and treatment of cancer. Another is the morbidity costs of cancer or the productivity losses due to illnesses. And the third is mortality costs, that is, the productivity loss due to premature death. The total cost estimated in 2004 was $189.9 billion (or $204.4 billion in 2006 dollars). Of that, $69.4 billion ($74.4 billion in 2006 dollars) was in direct medical costs. A large part of total costs is due also to morbidity ($16.9 billion, or $18.2 billion in 2006 dollars) and mortality ($103.5 billion, or $111.3 billion in 2006 dollars).

Total medical costs of cancer account for five percent of total healthcare expenditures in the nation, but in terms of Medicare expenditures, where the burden is concentrated, cancer patients account for about 10 percent of total costs. The trend in total cancer cost over time, comparing 1996 to 2005, shows a doubling in nominal numbers in less than 10 years. It is very important to consider the inflation factor so you know what these figures really mean. When that is done by normalizing everything into 2006 dollars, there is still a 40 percent increase in total cost. That means that the total cost of cancer is growing at a much faster pace than the general medical commodity inflation rate.

Examining the trend in direct medical costs of cancer alone shows an increase in nominal cost of about 75 percent and after adjustment for inflation of about 25 percent, again at a much higher pace than medical care inflation. Examining the distribution of total cost into the three types of costs shows an increasing percentage assigned to the direct medical costs component (from 29 percent in 1990 to 37 percent in 2004). This might be caused by two factors: the aging of the cancer population and new technology. This change in the distribution of costs to direct medical costs would probably be more pronounced in the elderly population as premature death costs would be much lower in this population.

The 1991 Medicare Current Beneficiary Survey found that Medicare reimbursement was $2,340 ($4,410 in 2006 dollars) annually on average per beneficiary for the entire Medicare population compared to $3,590 ($6,766 in 2006 dollars) for beneficiaries with cancer, about 1.5 times higher. A multivariate analysis compared cancer patients with patients with other chronic disease, for example, ischemic heart disease or COPD, and found that a diagnosis of cancer was associated strongly with higher Medicare expenditures (Stafford and Cyr, 1997).

Data from the 1995 Asset and Health Dynamics Study compared 2-year out-of-pocket expenses of patients 70 or older without cancer, with a history of cancer not currently being treated, and with cancer currently being treated. Adjusted annual out-of-pocket expenses for the groups were, respectively, $1,210, $1,450, and $1,880. Overall, the out-of-pocket expenditures for cancer patients were a great deal higher than for older persons without cancer. The costs were divided into four health-care service components: hospitalization, medication, outpatient visits, and home health care. Prescription medications and home health care services accounted for most of the higher costs. The finding that low-income elderly cancer patients spent about 27 percent of their annual income on medical costs, compared with only seven percent in the higher-income individuals is disturbing because it implies a much higher financial burden of cancer for a low-income elderly family (Langa et al., 2004).

Data from health management organizations (HMOs) during the period 1995 to 1998 were used to examine outpatient cancer drug costs for cancer patients of all ages. The drugs were divided into: antineoplastics; chemotherapy adjuncts (for example, growth factors or antiemetics); supportive drugs (for example, psychotherapy); and noncancer drugs. The cost of drugs administered in physicians' offices (mainly antineoplastics) rose from $5,137 to $8,170 over the 4 years. Outpatient pharmacy drug costs rose from $560 to $935. The major cost driver appeared to be the increase in technology represented by new anticancer agents (Halbert et al., 2002). I conclude from these data that even higher outpatient drug costs are likely in older persons as that would reflect the polypharmacy that we know is present in this age group.

So why am I talking about this? I want to direct your attention to Medicare Part D, the prescription drug program that started at the beginning of 2006. We know that as of June 2006 about 90 percent of Medicare beneficiaries already had drug coverage. There is a coverage gap (called the donut hole) in this program. When drug expenditures reach $2,250, patients are responsible for 100 percent of their outpatient prescription drug costs. At that point, it is essentially as though they have no insurance coverage until they have spent another $2,850, at which point the catastrophic feature of the plan kicks in. So this is the part that really concerns us.

It has been suggested that an extensive range of cancer drugs is now covered by Medicare Part D, and that this might result in lower out-of-pocket payments, because now patients do not have to pay out-of-pocket for the full costs of outpatient drugs (Bowman et al., 2006). Recall that we saw an unequal financial burden of cancer between the low- and high-income family. In the future, we would like to explore whether it is possible that Medicare Part D might be a policy that can reduce the disparity in financial burden between high- and low-income cancer families.

Relating now the data on drug costs that I have presented to the coverage gap I mentioned earlier, we saw average outpatient pharmacy drug costs of about $935 in 1998 or $1,278 in 2006 dollars for cancer patients of all ages. That is already very close to $2,250 where the coverage gap starts, and we know that in the elderly population outpatient drug costs will be a great deal higher. That means that it is possible that elderly cancer patients will reach the donut hole much earlier than most other elderly patients. These are things that I think are very important from a policy perspective but have not been studied so far.

Turning now to the economics of cancer prevention, many of the cost-effectiveness analyses of cancer screening rely on decision modeling because there is no information from clinical trials on screening in elderly people. Most studies have concluded that cancer screening is still cost effective in the elderly population, but there is some disagreement on the upper age for screening to be cost-effective. Some say mammography is cost-effective up to age 85; others say age 75 should be the upper age limit. The effectiveness of colorectal cancer screening is said to depend on age, comorbidity, and modality, with some variation in different population groups age 70 and over. Cervical cancer screening is said to be beneficial in the older population.

Coverage of cancer screening by Medicare is quite generous. Almost all the effective screening technologies are included, but the 20 percent coinsurance, which is waived for some tests, still applies to mammography, digital rectal exam (DRE), and colonoscopy, for example, and this can be an impediment for low-income populations. Studies of the impact of Medicare coverage on the uptake of cancer screening have shown that the economic factor is a common access barrier. However, even when Medicare covers screening thus removing the economic barrier, low rates of screening may persist in certain populations. For example, mammography screening benefits started in 1991, but a study of the rate of breast cancer screening before and after Medicare coverage found very little increase in utilization. The same study also found that an educational intervention plus Medicare payment seems to be a more effective way of increasing screening in this population (Breen et al., 1997).

Colonoscopy coverage for average-risk adults started in July 2001. Most reports in the literature support a subsequent increase in the rate of endoscopic colorectal cancer screening. Our own study found that even though this Medicare policy change alleviated the screening disparity between non-Hispanic whites and non-Hispanic blacks, the gap between Hispanic and non-Hispanic whites actually widened. This suggests that certain populations are not taking advantage of the Medicare benefit. We concluded that the lower catch-up rates might be because of a higher Hispanic poverty proportion and also a higher proportion of Hispanics without a usual source of care or even possibly cultural factors. Again, it seems that simply removing the economic barrier does not necessarily alleviate the problem of screening disparities (Shih et al., 2006).

New treatment technologies are being introduced, and we wonder about the implications for the cost-effectiveness of screening. If a new technology has good test characteristics, do we still need an annual schedule, or can we achieve the same level of effectiveness with a reduced schedule? Most of the studies of cost-effectiveness of mammography do not consider that the test characteristics are actually better in the older population, which implies that what we have discovered so far might actually underestimate the cost-effectiveness of screening in the older population.

We also need to look at the relationship between treatment innovation and the cost-effectiveness of prevention. There has been talk about chemoprevention and the use of pharmacogenomic tests, and these also would have an impact on the cost-effectiveness of screening and need to be considered in future studies.

Turning now to the economics of cancer treatment, the 2005 cancer trend progress report as displayed in Table 2-8 shows that lung, breast, colorectal, and prostate cancer plus lymphoma, these five cancers alone, consume about 50 percent of all Medicare cancer expenditures. An exami-

TABLE 2-8 Medicare Expenditures in the First Year of Diagnosis, by Cancer Type

Cancer Types	Percent of All Cancer Expenditures (%)	Per Capita (in 2006 dollars) (projected from 1996–1999 data)
Lung	13.3	26,572
Breast	11.2	11,834
Colorectal	11.7	26,034
Prostate	11.1	11,834
Lymphoma	6.3	23,129
Head/neck	4.4	19,364
Bladder	4.0	13,232
Leukemia	3.7	19,364
Ovary	3.1	39,589
Kidney	2.7	27,217

SOURCE: Adapted from Shih et al., 2006; adapted from NCI, 2005.

nation of per capita cancer expenditures reveals that ovarian cancer is very expensive when compared with breast and prostate cancer. In just the first year costs alone, then, we are talking about an average of about $22,000 per cancer patient.

Most studies of cancer-specific costs either use SEER-Medicare data or some kind of HMO/managed care data. We are fortunate to have the SEER-Medicare data because they are, so far, the best source of cost information for the elderly population. Studies usually stratify treatment cost data into initial, continuing, and terminal care phases. We often observe a U-shaped cost curve, meaning that there are higher costs in the initial and terminal phase and a lower cost in between. Most studies also use a case-control approach so that they can attribute costs to cancer rather than cite total costs, and studies also combine survival information to try to look at the long-term care costs of cancer patients. Most studies do not consider structural changes, which means that assessments of long-term costs do not consider possible innovations that might lead to better outcomes in the future.

Figure 2-14 displays breast cancer care cost data divided into phases for women in different age groups, using data from 1990 and 1991 (Taplin et al., 1995) and 1984–1990 (Riley et al., 1995) and updating all cost estimates to 2006 dollars. Regardless of the phase of care, there is a decrease in

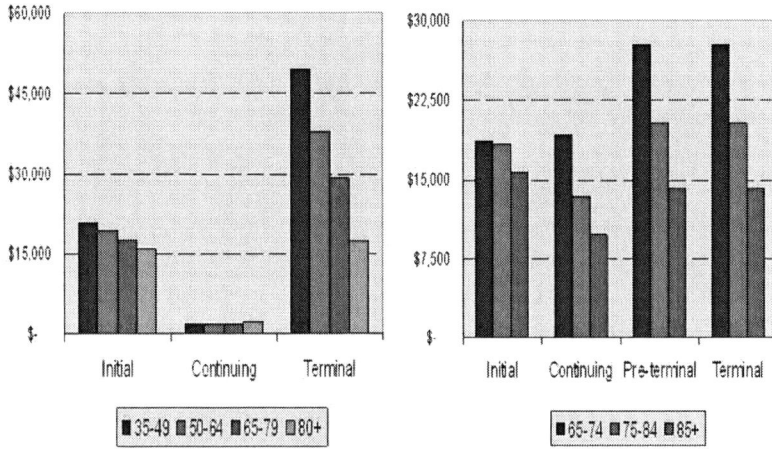

FIGURE 2-14 Cost of breast cancer treatment by age at various phases of care, in 2006 dollars.
SOURCE: Shih et al., 2006; modified from information from Taplin et al., 1995, and Riley et al., 1995.

trend of costs by age. This occurs comparing younger with older populations or within the older population itself. These earlier data show that elderly cancer patients were treated less aggressively than younger cancer patients, especially in the terminal care phase. More recent studies, using data from the 1990s, have found increasing use of chemotherapy in the 65 and over population; one study found that use of adjuvant chemotherapy increased from 7.4 percent in 1991 to 16.3 percent in 1999 (Giordano et al., 2006).

A similar pattern has been observed in other cancers. For example, a study by Earle and colleagues found increasing aggressiveness of care toward the end of life (Earle et al., 2004). All these reports suggest that as physicians are more willing to give chemotherapy to elderly cancer patients, we may see even higher treatment costs.

The American Cancer Society has predicted an oncology time bomb because of the technology advances that we are now seeing. Many of the new cancer drugs carry a very high price tag. In colorectal cancer, if you compare Avastin/Erbitux with the traditional 5FU plus Leucovorin regimen, the cost is about $21,000 to $30,000 higher. In lung cancer, the monthly cost of Iressa is $1,800, which must be taken for months or years, and $2,500 for Tarceva. The treatment of an early-stage breast cancer with Herceptin costs about $50,000 per year. So, the 20 percent coinsurance alone will cost a patient about $10,000 out-of-pocket.

The Medicare estimate using 1984–1990 data for total cost of care for breast cancer from diagnosis to death was $103,375 in 2006 dollars, but using the new data, we know that Herceptin alone costs $50,000 per year. These data tell us that just inflating previous cost estimates to a current dollar value is going to underestimate treatment costs because cancer care is inflating at a much faster rate than regular medical care. So there is a need to update the cost estimates to reflect the costs of newer cancer drugs.

Actually, an attempt has been made to project the impact of the newer drugs introduced using the Medicare Current Beneficiary Survey plus SEER data for 1992–2000 and various microsimulation models considering major advances in cancer and supportive care drugs from 2000 to 2004, among other scenarios. According to the projection with these new cancer drugs, $300 of cost will be added for every Medicare beneficiary, not just those with cancer, between 2005 and 2030, and the Medicare program will increase by $20 billion over the 2000 baseline. The incremental cost-effectiveness ratio for new treatments launched from 2000 to 2004 will be about $143,000. In this study, even under the most optimistic scenarios, Medicare program cost is unlikely to decline (Bhattacharya et al., 2005). These technologies have carried a high price tag and are not necessarily cost-effective to the system. Of course, there are demographic realities to consider. There is a competing risk; if people do not die of cancer, they will die of something else. So, in the future, there still will be an increasing Medicare expenditure whether or not we have the best cancer treatments in the world.

The clinical management of older patients has become more complex. There are many factors that contribute to a possibly higher cost of adverse events in elderly people. Normal hematopoietic and nervous system, heart, mucosa, and other tissues become more vulnerable to chemotherapy with aging. There is a higher incidence of depression and anemia, and polypharmacy or even the behavior of cancer itself may increase the risk of adverse events, and these events increase the need (and the costs) for supportive care products, such as growth factors and EPO.

Medicare data from 1996–1999 show that hospice care costs $27,917 in the last year of life of cancer patients compared with costs of $29,905 for cancer patients who are not in hospice, so early studies concluded that hospice may be cost neutral or cost saving for Medicare (Campbell et al.,

2004). But use of hospice seems to be negatively related to the aggressiveness of care (Earle et al., 2004). Treatment innovations, then, may lead to decreasing use of hospice and loss of any savings.

The Medicare Modernization Act changed Medicare reimbursement for chemotherapy drugs from average wholesale price to average sales price plus 6 percent, reducing the profits of oncology practices. We know that some physicians, including oncologists, react to financial incentives; thus, reduction of reimbursement may cause a shift of care to hospital outpatient departments. A recent study of Medicare cancer patients from 1995 to 1998 also discovered that oncologists react by prescribing better reimbursed drugs, although reimbursement does not seem to affect the decision to start chemotherapy (Jacobson et al., 2006). If we believe that the more costly drugs are the better ones, then we may be creating a disparity by a different payment system.

Medicare Part D now covers oral hormonal cancer drugs. Previously, oral antiandrogens were underprescribed for prostate cancer in part because of lack of insurance coverage, although also because antiandrogens have not been shown to confer substantial survival advantage. With Part D coverage, we may see increasing use of oral hormonal therapy to the extent that some patients might actually substitute antiandrogens for regular care. We need to look into that.

The different coinsurance and scope of coverage between the existing Part B (20 percent coinsurance) and new Part D (25 percent coinsurance and a donut hole) Medicare reimbursement for drugs injects another source of confusion into the picture. We do not yet know how the potential distortion of care by this economic factor will play out. We should take a careful look at this issue, but it is not clear when CMS will release the data to researchers.

The cost of treatment-related late complications has not been studied in the literature. Many of the complications, such as lymphedema, pain, fatigue, and depression, are likely to be even more prevalent in the elderly population, either because of the biology of aging or, for example, because some breast cancer patients treated 20 years ago with more radical surgery are now accumulating in the older survivor populations. So those patients are in the system now, but we just do not know how costly they are to the system.

The cost of informal caregiving is higher for cancer patients amounting to 3.1 more hours per week or about $1,200 per patient per year (Hayman et al., 2001). Health-care costs for informal caregiver have not been well studied. The focus has been on productivity loss by informal caregivers, but the higher rate of depression and lower self-perceived health reported by informal caregivers might translate to higher health-care costs for informal caregivers. The greater prevalence of comorbidities in the elderly cancer population might also increase the caregivers' burden. And the unequal financial burden for high- versus low-income cancer families might also apply to the informal caregiver population, as we know that poor families are less likely to use any kind of formal care for cancer patients because they can not afford to.

Finally, as I said at the beginning, I would like to end with a few brief comments on supply-side considerations. We know that health economics studies have found that outcomes might vary by different organizational types (for-profit versus not-for-profit). There have been several types of new organizations developed in response to financial pressures in cancer care. Physician oncology networks have sprung up to provide carve-out oncology care, and some managed care systems have started to use capitated or disease management type models for cancer care, although these have not been very successful. Under the Medicare Modernization Act we might see community oncologists contracting with specialty pharmacies to cut down on oncology drug costs (Reeder and Gordon, 2006). Very few studies have examined the relationship between organizational factors and patient outcomes or quality of cancer care, so those are also studies that we need to look into.

There are a number of reasons for concern about the future adequacy of the oncology workforce, including the projected increase in cancer incidence and prevalence in the growing older population matched with the stable number of oncologists in training; the increasing numbers of cancer survivors and their needs for long-term follow-up and care; and reduced Medicare payment as a disincentive for some trainees to enter the oncology subspecialty.

At this point, do we have any evidence of a workforce shortage? The answer is yes. A 2002 American Society for Therapeutic Radiology and Oncology (ASTRO) workforce study found a significant shortage in the radiation oncology workforce. For oncology nursing, the shortage has also been documented, and the ASCO partnership with AAMC to study the supply of general medical oncologists was referred to earlier. We also know there is a shortage in the physician workforce in rural areas. So we can project that it is going to be even more problematic for cancer patients in rural areas because specialists such as oncologists tend to practice in urban communities.

In summary, then, we know there is a trend toward more aggressive cancer treatment in the elderly population, and we know that this is going to translate into a higher cost of caring for those patients. Studies need to be done to update earlier cost estimates to reflect technology advances because we know that just adjusting by inflation is not enough. We also need to reevaluate the disease burden and the cost-effectiveness of treatment to account for the unique physiologic characteristics of the elderly cancer population. We need to assess the effects of Medicare Part D and the Medicare Modernization Act on practice patterns, costs, and the disparities in financial burdens between high- and low-income cancer families. And finally, we need to examine strategies to address workforce shortages, such as using telemedicine or incentive programs to attract physicians to rural communities.

Dr. Yancik: Thank you very much for that abundant information and a great talk, well delivered. I do not know if anybody else agrees, but what we are facing in terms of costs seems overwhelming.

Dr. Foley: When ASCO studied physicians' behaviors toward end-of-life care, they reported that they were not reimbursed to do it in an outpatient setting, and, therefore, did not do it. In discussing the proposed change in reimbursement for drugs, oncologists claimed that they had used the profits from drugs at average wholesale price to provide care for patients, to provide support. Now that drug profits have been reduced, they no longer will be able to provide that support, which will, in fact, affect their ability to care for complicated patients with complicated regimens, and, therefore, shift those patients back into a hospital setting. So I think it is all sort of a domino effect that could easily take place.

Ann O'Mara, Program Director, Community Clinical Oncology Program, National Cancer Institute: Research Issues: I will be talking about what NCI is supporting regarding cancer in older persons in the extramural community. This means all the projects that are brought forward to the NCI for peer review, both investigator initiated and K awards. Also, I will discuss what the cooperative groups are doing in terms of the elderly population, because that is where a good amount of resources are.

What we support responds to four overarching clinical problems: the underutilization of prevention strategies within the elderly cancer population; late diagnosis in that population; undertreatment; and, finally, defining the older person—is that a 68-year-old who just ran the marathon yesterday or a 68-year-old with several comorbidities and a stroke? The definition is important to our cooperative groups and when accruing patients to our treatment trials when we specify patients must be age 65 or over. We are getting better at listing some of our comorbidities and refining that, but it still is quite a struggle.

A search of the Computer Retrieval of Information on Scientific Projects (CRISP) public database of all funded projects for cancer in the older population yielded 19 relevant projects: 12 were investigator initiated, either RO1s, R21s, or the small RO3s; five were K mechanisms, specifically focused on developing a career in working with the older population, and two in the U mechanism, which were not cooperative groups but cooperative agreements. And there were seven different foci of these projects: four of them were focused on novel treatment or dosing schedules unique to the older population; four on prevention and screening, of which two were really comparing screening in cancer patients for cancer versus noncancer patients and screening for hypertension, diabetes, and so on. I am curious what the outcomes of those might have shown, whether we are screening better in the cancer population than in other chronic disease populations. Three projects focused on health services utilization; two on short- and long-term sequelae from cancer treatment; two on comorbidities; two on treatment utilization; and two on patient preferences and decision making about whether or not to take chemotherapy.

When I examined how our investigators are going about pursuing these studies, I discovered, as you have previously heard, that most were secondary analyses employing the SEER-Medicare database. All four of the novel treatment or dosing schedules were clinical trials (and these were outside of the cooperative groups that I will cover later). The prevention and screening studies were secondary analyses (except for one or two that were prospective observational), as were all the health services utilization studies. There was one clinical trial focusing on ameliorating fatigue in cancer survivors over age 65 in the short- and long-term sequelae group, and the rest of the projects were either observational or secondary analyses. So that is the state of our current support of our investigator pool. I should caution you, however, that there are limitations to this search of CRISP, most notably that it yielded projects that were focused on the older population, and there may be many others that include older people in their particular trials.

With respect to clinical trials and the cooperative groups, more than

50 percent of our adult cancer population is over 65, but only about 2.5 percent of our total U.S. adult cancer population accrue to NCI-supported trials, and less than one percent of the U.S. cancer population over 65 accrue to these NCI-supported trials. So the generalizability to older people of findings from our clinical trials is suspect at best.

But, when I examined our disease treatment trials as well as our prevention and symptom management trials, I found some improvement. In our disease treatment trials, between 2001 and 2005, 30 percent of adult patients were over 65. Of these, over 80 percent were in the 65 to 70 group. Then, about 38 percent of our adult patients in prevention and symptom management trials were over age 65. So, that is somewhat reassuring. Nevertheless, the fact remains that we are only accruing about 2.5 percent of the adult population to our treatment trials.

I should point out that the NCI has no information on industry-sponsored studies. We are not given information on the age of those patients unless we are also cosponsoring that study. And we do not collect information on institutional treatment trials at NCI-designated cancer centers. If you remember, our project enrollment is gender and ethnicity and race, not on age. So that is the information that we are collecting from our cancer centers.

What are the barriers to enrolling elderly people? It goes back to how we define them, and it is related to our trial eligibility and how we list our comorbidities. We also have physician bias in terms of patients being eligible. Do they believe that they are eligible and appropriate for the trial? There is patient and family bias and myths that patients and families have about accruing to clinical trials. Social support that would encourage enrollment of the elderly cancer population in trials is a problem. Finally, what we know about referral patterns to cancer centers, as well as what we have learned about cancer within Medicare, suggests barriers to access to clinical trials.

Currently, the NCI is sponsoring 12 cooperative group trials from phase 1 through phase 3, of which half are in acute myelogenous leukemia and the rest divided among lung (nonsmall cell), breast, brain, and genito-urinary cancer.

So, that summarizes where we are in cancer in the older population at the NCI through our R and K awards and where we are with our national clinical trials network, both from the Division of Cancer Treatment and more or less the Community Clinical Oncology Program of symptom management and prevention trials.

Dr. Ganz: Did you look at the Institute for Nursing Research portfolio or perhaps the NIA? I just wondered if any might be hiding over there.

Dr. O'Mara: That is a good question, and I did not. One could also look at the NIMH, because they do support some of these areas there.

Dr. Ganz: But when we hear our portfolio analyses at the Board of Scientific Advisors and they want us to support a request for applications, they say 34 projects is low, and you have only 19.

Dr. Yancik, Research Issues: I have worked in the NIA for 15 years. After 5 years in the NIA Office of the Director I had the opportunity to transfer into the extramural program to develop research on aging and cancer. I developed two program announcements immediately (1996), and then I convened a group of people to give me advice (1997). I am still working on the kinds of projects listed in Table 2-9. As you can see, coverage of our general areas of interest is broad.

The NIA was established in 1974. In terms of its size and funding, probably it is midway within the spectrum of institutes. There was then and there is now much social concern about the aging population and a great deal of interest in health services for older persons that helped to build the NIA. A 1971 White House Conference on Aging spurred it on; there was a House Select Committee on Aging convened and chaired by Representative Claude D. Pepper. The programs of the institute include biology

TABLE 2-9 NIA Priority Areas for Integration of Aging/Cancer Research

- Age-related factors in development of tumors in older persons
- Time and its importance in developing cancer in a person's life span
- Aggressive tumor behavior in the aged patient
- Pharmacology of aging and cancer—antitumor drug alterations
- Prognostic indicators for patient evaluation and workup
- Comorbidity, previous illness, and disabilities in older cancer patients
- Occurrence of multiple primary tumors in the elderly
- Cancer survivorship—need long-term data on older cancer survivors
- Access issues for older patients, their families, and physicians
- Use generic age-related issues as in breast and prostate program announcements (PAs)

SOURCE: Yancik, 1997b.

of aging, behavioral and social science, neuroscience and neuropsychology, geriatrics and clinical gerontology, and the intramural program (Baltimore). The Geriatrics and Clinical Gerontology Program has research centers. They are called the Older American Independence Centers and are named after Representative Claude D. Pepper. Research topics include frailty prevention, menopause, health and longevity, osteoporosis and musculoskeletal disorders, falls prevention, geriatric syndromes, cardiovascular disorders, and cancer and aging. There are about 9–10 studies ongoing at any one time. They do not have to recompete every 5 years.

The Cancer Research Initiatives that I initiated in conjunction with colleagues in other institutes include integrating aging and cancer research (R01s); aging, race, and ethnicity in prostate cancer; aging women and breast cancer; NCI clinical trials cooperative groups; studies on older patients; aging and risk factors for multiple primary tumors; cancer pharmacology and treatment in older patients; bioimaging techniques for early prostate cancer; long-term survivors research initiatives; interdisciplinary studies in genetic epidemiology of cancer; late medical effects of cancer treatment in older women; and diagnostic cancer imaging and radiation therapy in older patients. These have been issued as program announcements or requests for applications.

Cancer pharmacology and treatment in older patients was the topic of a program announcement. Aging and risk factors for multiple primary tumors is one of my major interests. The NCI clinical trials cooperative groups studies on older cancer patients has generated the CALGB cancer clinical trial for older women and companion studies, as I mentioned. We have joined with the NCI for long-term survivors research initiatives. The interdisciplinary studies in genetic epidemiology and diagnostic cancer imaging and radiation therapy RFAs were initiated by the NCI; we joined as a dual assignment for some grants. We achieved a major goal by issuing the aging, race, and ethnicity in prostate cancer RFA.

To examine the pharmacology of aging and cancer the NCI is pursuing studies on dosage, administration, and special monitoring needs of older persons with cancer; treatment considerations factoring in changes in body composition and organ function, drug tolerance, and drug-drug interaction; relationship of drug interventions or combination therapies as they occur in combination with age-associated comorbidities (and in comorbid disease-free patients); and interaction with older persons' own use of medications and other prescribed and over-the-counter medications.

The relationship of drug interventions or combination therapies as they occur in combination with age-associated comorbidities is very important. Comorbidity and the influence of frailty on the course of cancer patient management are so important for the early detection of primary cancer or recurrence. The NIA and the NCI held a large workshop to explore the role of NCI-designated cancer centers for integrating aging and cancer research in 2001. We convened plenary sessions and seven working groups for 2 1/2 days. We had approximately 120 participants. I worked with the cancer center branch staff in putting together the initiative under which eight cancer centers received awards in August 2003. This a $26-million project shared equally by the NCI and the NIA. I would like to share the NIA/NCI workshop report with you. It can be found at http://www.nia.nih.gov/ResearchInformation/ConferencesandMeetings/WorkshopReport.

Thanks for the opportunity to present these aging and cancer research efforts that have developed.

Dr. Jerome Yates, Research Issues: I am going to talk both about the American Cancer Society (ACS) research program and a little bit about our advocacy efforts, things that we can do to try to enhance progress. There are activities inside of the ACS that are not directly related to research activities. We have health promotions that are largely public education and other efforts involving our collaboration with the NCI. We are funding one of the navigator research sites, and we are also funding the training and the evaluation for the NCI-supported navigator activities. We think that, in the end, this will help us optimize our programs and also enhance our relationships with the NCI.

We do a great deal of public education, and we target that to some extent. We operate our National Cancer Information Center, a 24-hour, 7-day a week telephone access cancer help line. On the epidemiological front, the ACS annual *Cancer Facts and Figures* publication is widely used. The cohort studies (Cancer Prevention Studies 1 and 2–CPS-1 and 2) have looked at tobacco smoking and cancer in the past and cancer and obesity more recently. There is another study in the works, CPS-3, that will be an epidemiological (prospective cohort) study that will involve collecting biologic materials and seek to better understand the relationships among lifestyle and behavioral, environmental, and genetic factors that cause or prevent cancer. Our Behavioral Research Center is largely focused on survivor and patient care studies now, but it will be looking at provider and patient decision making in the future.

From 1998 to 2007, we have funded eight training grants at the masters of science (M.S.) and doctorate (Ph.D.) levels, eight basic science laboratory grants, two screening grants for colorectal cancer, two on comorbidity, two on cancer care, one on pain management, and one on quality of life in lymphoma at a total of $7,526,000. The M.S. and Ph.D. training grants are for nurses and social workers. The basic science grants are related to aging studies at the cellular or basic level.

Our advocacy activities are going to focus a great deal on access to health care, both the legislation, it is hoped, for universal health care and how the regulations are written. We have been trying to get the CMS to perform a chronic disease, cancerlike demonstration project, and I think that some coordinated effort from a variety of organizations might, in fact, help that to come about. In the targeted research area, although this is not elderly research, we have set aside $500,000 for pilot projects for palliative care research. This is largely to generate data so that people will have enough information to submit RO1s. We received 130 applications for this; there is a great deal of interest out there. We also set aside $1 million for health policy research, which is going to be focused, we think, in areas that are relevant to the mission of the ACS. We have formed a coalition with the heart and diabetes associations to look specifically at obesity and exercise activities and generally at disease prevention. Needless to say, we are part of a large group of organizations that are trying to get more funding for the NIH.

We have already talked about the changing demographics today. Here we need more public education (including caregivers) and I think some social solutions. National data showed in 1995 that 46 percent of women over 65 were widowed. There clearly will be many widows in the coming decades. The living arrangements are such that men are living with their wives, and widows are living alone or with nonfamily. Social support for those that are living alone will be needed, as many have limited social activity and insecurity about any source of assistance if needed. And they have greater levels of depression, poor adjustment to illness, and increased relative risk of mortality if they are isolated compared to those with support.

The economics are not reassuring. In 2006, there will be five workers for each retiree and Medicare will be 8 percent of GDP. In 2030, there will be three workers per retiree and Medicare is projected at 13 percent of GDP. It certainly looks as though we are going to have some big problems in terms of how we finance these programs.

Now, I would like to briefly touch on the Value of Health and Longevity study and what that tells us about looking at the economics of these issues (Murphy and Topel, 2006). We have already been addressing the productivity issues, and there are many studies looking at the cost of care at the end of life. This study examined the dollars that are spent for different age groups; it considered the individuals' willingness to pay to maintain health and used the values ascribed to that willingness to assign values to health improvements. From 1970 to 2000, improved life expectancy added $3.2 trillion per year to national wealth (or about half of GDP), and a permanent 1 percent reduction in mortality from cancer was calculated to have a value of $500 billion. This was not the result of increased productivity from avoidable mortality. For individuals, significant personal values were calculated for a 10 percent reduction in cancer mortality at all ages even including into the 70s and 80s. The social value of health improvements will improve with increased population growth, increased capital incomes (unless there are cuts in social programs), and increased growth in the component for the older population even with medical conditions.

There have been a couple of studies lately that have highlighted the fact that the common cancers in elderly people are heterogeneous and that we are not likely to have single specific treatments for them as we do for chronic myelocytic leukemia or gastrointestinal stromal tumors. That emphasizes the importance of detecting the disease early and treating patients with surgery to the extent that we can. There may at some point be tests such as the PSA or the like that will help with that.

A recent Agency for Healthcare Research and Quality (AHRQ) report noted the great increase in lumpectomies for treatment of breast cancer. Because half of breast cancer is in elderly people, these older women will be receiving treatment in the outpatient setting and then will be going home. At that point, someone will have to care for them, and the education to do this is not in place. One can only imagine some of the problems that occur as a result of this deficit.

So where should we go in the future? I think we need to have better early detection programs. We need to be able to categorize comorbidities with some consistency. Palliative care is clearly important. Individuals are going to need to be liberated from institutions, hospitals, and nursing homes, but if we do that we need the support systems in place to take care of these individuals when they are outside of these institutions. And there has to be a better way of monitoring the quality of care in these situations. At the moment, there is no infrastructure to do this. So we need some changes in health policy. We need to think about the caregivers; we need to be able to train them and provide them with adequate backup and support. We need incentives for families to take care of the patient, so all of this is not just out-of-pocket care, and the ACS will think about modifying some of its traditional supportive programs, such as Reach to Recovery, to try to fill some of these niches.

Dr. Ganz: Just to that last point, in California, because of the managed care situation, we have been seeing mostly outpatient procedures for a long time. I have been seeing women who have never had any education about lymphedema-protective activities. They had not been given any guidance or counseling. In the old days, when they were in the hospital for 5 to 7 days, and there was not much going on, the nurses did a great deal of education, and the Reach to Recovery volunteer came by. So what has happened? I think there is such a void there now that there is a real need for your types of programs.

Dr. Yates: Yes, we need to restructure the Reach to Recovery Program. We ought to be talking about different kinds of messages. Formerly, there was a fair amount of physical therapy along with psychosocial support. Now there is some psychosocial support, but we really could be conveying better educational messages, and I think that is what we need to think about doing.

Dr Ferrell: The American Cancer Society could make a great contribution by creating a "preparing to care for someone you love with cancer" program, where family members could come in and learn about caring throughout the whole trajectory of cancer care.

Dr. Yates: We are developing a curriculum for the Navigator Program that addresses helping people, understanding what questions to ask, and what needs to be emphasized. We could address caregiving in cancer in a similar way and try to develop a curriculum to address the important issues. I hope I could call on some of you to participate in that activity.

Ms. Boyle: I think there are programs that are trying to do it. The problem is they do not publish, but if there was a way to have a workshop to look at best practices, some of those who have tried educational interventions could describe their work. I know in Australia, there is a large breast care nurse contingent within oncology nursing; it would be interesting to see their curriculum.

Dr. Yates: Agreed, although they have socialized medicine, and that makes it much easier to incorporate these things into the health-care system.

Dr. Matrisian: On the research side, the NCI/NIA joint centers seem a sensible idea. So, three years in, how are they working?

Dr. Yancik: The rationale behind the initiative was to give enough resources to the grantees so they could build an aging and cancer component into their core grant or its equivalent and ultimately obtain continued funding. They have just entered their fourth year. The last two annual meetings have been extremely useful with good attendance, including both the NCI and NIA directors. Those involved feel they are all under one roof as part of the group. Yes, it remains to be seen whether or not they will all be successful, but everybody seems to be working as hard as they can and are involved in generating research support in the crosscutting areas they selected.

Dr. Foley: We did not talk today about how the Centers for Disease Control and Prevention (CDC), with the state plans, are addressing this issue. And the most marginalized populations that would be effected by this are clearly those who do not have access, and that would be our minority populations. We did not talk about Native Americans. We did not talk about African Americans in any great detail, and then there is a prison population who are aging and have cancer. So, there are three disparity populations that I think need some coverage on this issue, who get marginalized to begin with, and then, if they are elderly, get even more marginalized in the health care system. We should also think about our illegal immigrants.

Mr. Kean: I learned a great deal today that was very helpful to me. At the end of November, the National Partners for Comprehensive Cancer Control are convening to talk about phase 4 of the leadership institutes and state plan implementation that begins in early 2007, and I made a number of notes today on things that ought to be considered. I will carry the message back about some of the issues you put on the table today.

Dr. Yates: One of the problems about the state cancer plans, as you know, is most of them did not get funded. But the ACS will use the report card for the states, have the divisions support better pain management in those respective states, and use their clout to try to change legislation and regulations in the individual states.

In terms of disparities, the Navigator Program was actually designed to address the disparity issue, and, using unpublished data from the American College of Surgeons National Cancer Database, Elizabeth Ward has compared educational levels of cancer patients with survival data and found that mortality is inversely related to education level. Education level is more important than income in terms of determining survival, and this is not just true for cancer.

We think the Navigator Program will help these people navigate the system better than they would if they were alone. We also are looking at establishing a national vice president for disparities, because one of the internal complaints that we have had is that, although we talk about doing something about disparities, we have not done a great deal so far.

Ms. Boyle: In terms of the earlier comment about culture, I just tried to review the literature on breast and prostate cancer specific to African Americans in getting ready to do a talk in South Carolina, and there is very little. So it is another area where there is a big question mark.

Dr. Robinson: There is a website by the Office of Minority Health Resource Center, HtmlResAnchor www.omhrc.gov, that has information from the different racial and ethnic groups on different health topics, including cancer, with statistics on various cancers in the major racial and ethnic minority groups. I do not recall specifically if there is detail about age groups.

Dr. Silliman: The age structure of many of these minority populations, such as Hispanics, is younger. Only about five percent of older breast cancer patients with early-stage disease are African American, and this sort of thing makes the numbers problematic for studies in one geographic location. So you need to have integrated health systems or take advantage of SEER-Medicare data. Those are some of the challenges, not to say it is not really important. In integrated health plans such as Kaiser where people have uniform coverage, the disparities are nonexistent.

Dr. Moses: Concluding Remarks and Adjourn: I would like to thank all the speakers and the discussants. It has been a good day, and when it is written up I think it will make a good report. Many thanks to all of you.

References

Balducci, L. 2003. Review: New paradigms for treating elderly patients with cancer: The comprehensive geriatric assessment and guidelines for supportive care. *Journal of Supportive Oncology* 1(2):31.

Bhattacharya, J., B. Shang, C. K. Su, and D. P. Goldman. 2005. Technological advances in cancer and future spending by the elderly. *Health Affairs* 24(suppl 2):W5R53-W5R66.

Bowman, J., A. Rousseau, D. Silk, and C. Harrison. 2006. Access to cancer drugs in Medicare Part D: Formulary placement and beneficiary cost sharing in 2006. *Health Affairs* 25(5):1240-1248.

Boyle, D. A. 2001. Cancer in the elderly. In *Oncology nursing series. 2nd ed.*, edited by R. Fink and R. Gates R. Philadelphia, PA: Hanley and Belfus.

Breen, N., E. J. Feuer, S. Depuy, and J. Zapka. 1997. Effect of Medicare reimbursement for screening mammography on utilization and payment. National Cancer Institute Breast Cancer Screening Consortium. *Public Health Reports* 112(5):423-432.

Bynum, J. P. W., J. B. Braunstein, P. Sharkey, K. Haddad, and A. W. Wu. 2005. The influence of health status, age, and race on screening mammography in elderly women. *Archives of Internal Medicine* 165:2083-2088.

Campbell, D. E., J. Lynn, T. A. Louis, and L. R. Shugarman. 2004. Medicare program expenditures associated with hospice use. *Annals of Internal Medicine* 140(4):269-277.

Casarett, D., R. Crowley, C. Stevenson, S. Xie, and J. Teno. 2005. Making difficult decisions about hospice enrollment: What do patients and families want to know? *Journal of the American Geriatrics Society* 53(2):249-254.

Catt, S., M. Blanchard, J. Addington-Hall, M. Zis, B. Blizard, and M. King. 2005. The development of a questionnaire to assess the attitudes of older people to end-of-life issues (AEOLI). *Palliative Medicine* 19(5):397-401.

Dacal, K., S. M. Serelka, and S. L. Greenspan. 2006. Quality of life in prostate cancer patients taking androgen deprivation therapy. *Urologic Oncology* 24(5):458-459.

Demark-Wahnfried, W., B. M. Pinto,, and E. R. Gritz. 2006. Promoting health and physical function among cancer survivors: Potential for prevention and questions that remain. *Journal of Clinical Oncology* 24(32):5125-5131.

Earle, C. C., H. F. Burstein, E. P. Winer, and J. C. Weeks. 2003. Quality of non-breast cancer health maintenance among elderly breast cancer survivors. *Journal of Clinical Oncology* 21(8):1447-1451.

Earle, C. C., B. A. Neville, M. B. Landrum, J. Z. Ayanian, S. D. Block, and J. C. Weeks. 2004. Trends in the aggressiveness of cancer care near the end of life. *Journal of Clinical Oncology* 22(2):315-321.

Emanuel, E. J., Y. Young-Xu, N. G. Levinsky, G. Gazelle, O. Saynina, and S. Ash. 2003. Chemotherapy use among Medicare beneficiaries at the end of life. *Annals of Internal Medicine* 138(8):639-643.

Enger, S. M., S. S. Thwin,, D. S. Bulst, T. Field, F. Frost, A. M. Geiger, T. L. Lash, M. Prout, M. U. Yood, F. Wei, and R. A. Silliman. 2006. Breast cancer treatment of older women in integrated health care settings. *Journal of Clinical Oncology* 24(27):4369-4370.

Ferrell, B., R. Virani, S. Smith, and G. Juarez. 2003. The role of oncology nursing to ensure quality care for cancer survivors: A report commissioned by the National Cancer Policy Board and the Institute of Medicine. *Oncology Nursing Forum* 30(1):E1-E11.

Giordano, S. H., Z. Duan, Y. F. Kuo, G. N. Hortobagyi, and J. S. Goodwin. 2006. Use and outcomes of adjuvant chemotherapy in older women with breast cancer. *Journal of Clinical Oncology* 24(18):2697-2979.

Given, B., C. Given, F. Azzouz, and M. Stommel. 2001. Physical functioning of elderly cancer patients prior to diagnosis and following initial treatment. *Nursing Research* 50(4):222-232.

Goldstein, N. E., and R. S. Morrison. 2005. The intersection between geriatrics and palliative care: A call for a new research agenda. *Journal of the American Geriatrics Society* 53(9):1593-1598.

Goodwin, J. S., W. C. Hunt, and J. H. Samet. 1991. A population-based study of functional status and social support networks of elderly patients newly diagnosed with cancer. *Archives of Internal Medicine* 151(2):366-370.

Halbert, R. J., C. Zaher, S. Wade, J. Malin, G. D. Lawless, and R. W. Dubois. 2002. Outpatient cancer drug costs: Changes, drivers, and the future. *Cancer* 94(4):1142-1150.

Hayman, J. A., K. M. Langa, M. U. Kabeto, S. J. Katz, S. M. DeMonner, M. E. Chernew, M. B. Slavin, and A. M. Fendrick. 2001. Estimating the cost of informal caregiving for elderly patients with cancer. *Journal of Clinical Oncology* 19(13):3219-3225.

Heflin, M. T., K. I. Pollak, B. G. Kuchibhatla, and E. Z. Oddone. 2006. The impact of health status on physicians' intentions to offer cancer screening to older women. *Journal of Gerontology Series A: Biological Sciences and Medical Sciences* 61:844-850.

Hurria, A., M. S. Lachs, H. J. Cohen, H. B. Muss, and A. B. Kornblith. 2006. Geriatric assessment for oncologists: Rationale and future directions. *Critical Reviews in Oncology/Hematology* 59(3):211-217.

Hutchins, L. F., J. M. Unger, J. J. Crowley, C. A. Coltman, Jr., and K. S. Albain. 1999. Underrepresentation of patients 65 years of age or older in cancer-treatment trials. *New England Journal of Medicine* 341(27):2061-2067.

Hwang, S. S., V. T. Chang, J. Cogswell, S. Srinivas, and B. Kasimis. 2003. Knowledge and attitudes toward end-of-life care in veterans with symptomatic metastatic cancer. *Palliative & Supportive Care* 1(3):221-230.

Jacobson, M., A. J. O'Malley, C. C. Earle, J. Pakes, P. Gaccione, and J. P. Newhouse. 2006. Does reimbursement influence chemotherapy treatment for cancer patients? *Health Affairs* 25(2):437-443.

Keating, N. L., M. B. Landrum, E. Guadagnoli, E. P. Winer, and J. Z. Ayanian. 2006. Factors related to underuse of surveillance mammography among breast cancer survivors. *Journal of Clinical Oncology* 24(1):85-94.

Khatcheressian, J. L., A. C. Wolff, T. J. Smith, E. Grunfeld, H. B. Muss, V. G. Vogel, F. Halberg, M. R. Somerfield, and N. E. Davidson. 2006. American Society of Clinical Oncology 2006 update of the breast cancer follow-up and management guidelines in the adjuvant setting. *Journal of Clinical Oncology* 24:5091-5097.

Knols, R., N. K. Aaronson, D. Uebelhart, J. Fransen, and G. Aufdemkampe. 2005. Physical exercise in cancer patients during and after medical treatment: A systematic review of randomized and controlled clinical trials. *Journal of Clinical Oncology* 23(15):3830-3842.

Langa, K. M., A. M. Fendrick, M. E. Chernew, M. U. Kabeto, K. L. Paisley, and J. A. Hayman. 2004. Out-of-pocket health-care expenditures among older Americans with cancer. *Value in Health: The Journal of the International Society for Pharmacoeconomics and Outcomes Research* 7(2):186-194.

Lash, T. L., R. A. Silliman, E. Guadagnoli, and V. Mor. 2000. The effect of less than definitive care on breast carcinoma recurrence and mortality. *Cancer* 89(8):1739-1747.

Lash, T. L., K. Clough-Gorr, and R. A. Silliman. 2005. Reduced rates of cancer-related worries and mortality associated with guideline surveillance after breast cancer therapy. *Breast Cancer Research and Treatment* 89:61-67.

Lee, S. J., K. Lindquist, M. R. Segal, and K. E. Covinsky. 2006. Development and validation of a prognostic index for 4-year mortality in older adults. *Journal of the American Medical Association* 295:801-808.

Lunney, J. R., J. Lynn, D. J. Foley, S. Lipson, and J. M. Guralnik. 2003. Patterns of functional decline at the end of life. *Journal of the American Medical Association* 289(18):2387-2392.

Mandelblatt, J. S., C. B. Schechter, K. R. Yabroff, W. Lawrence, J. Dignam, M. Extermann, S. Fox, G. Orosz, R. Silliman, J. Cullen, L. Balducci, Breast Cancer in Older Women Research Consortium. 2005. Toward optimal screening strategies for older women. Costs, benefits, and harms of breast cancer screening by age, biology, and health status. *Journal of General Internal Medicine* 20(6):55203.

McQuellon, R. P., H. T. Thaler, D. Cella, and D. H. Moore. 2006. Quality of life (QOL) outcomes from a randomized trial of cisplatin versus cisplatin plus paclitaxel in advanced cervical cancer: a Gynecologic Oncology Group study. *Gynecologic Oncology* 101(2):296-304.

Murphy, K., and R. H. Topel. 2006. The value of health and longevity. *Journal of Political Economy* 114:871-904.

NCI (National Cancer Institute). 2005. *Cancer trend progress report.* http://progressreport.cancer.gov (accessed February 6, 2007).

Oncology Nursing Society, and Geriatric Oncology Consortium. 2004. Oncology Nursing Society and Geriatric Oncology Consortium joint position on cancer care in the older adult. *Oncology Nursing Forum* 31(3):489-490

Partridge, A. H., J. Avorn, P. S. Wang, and E. P. Winer. 2002. Adherence to therapy with oral antineoplastic agents. *Journal of the National Cancer Institute* 94(9):652-661.

Pignato, S., S. DePlacido, R. Biamonte, G. Scambia, G. DiVagno, G. Colucci, A. Febbraro, M. Farinaccio, A. V. Lombardi, L. Manzione, G. Carteni, M. Nardi, S. Canese, M. R. Valerio, A. Matteis, B. Massidda, G. Gasparini, M. DiMaio, C. Pisano, and F. Perrone. 2006. Residual neurotoxicity in ovarian cancer patients in clinical remission after first-line chemotherapy with carboplatin and paclitaxel: The Multicenter Italian Trial in Ovarian Cancer (MITO-4) Retrospective Study. *BioMed Central Cancer* 6:5.

Reeder, C. E., and D. Gordon. 2006. Managing oncology costs. *American Journal of Managed Care* 12(suppl 1):S3-S16.

Riley, G. F., A. L. Potosky, J. D. Lubitz,, and L. G. Kessler. 1995. Medicare payments from diagnosis to death for elderly cancer patients by stage at diagnosis. *Medical Care* 33(8):828-841.

Shih, Y. C., L. Zhao, and L. S. Etting. 2006. Does Medicare coverage of colonoscopy reduce racial/ethnic disparities in cancer screening among the elderly? *Health Affairs* 25(4):1153-1162.

Smith, B. D., C. P. Gross, G. L. Smith, D. H. Galusha, J. E. Bekelman, and B. G. Haffty. 2006. Effectiveness of radiation therapy for older women with early breast cancer. *Journal of the National Cancer Institute* 98:681-690.

Smith, M. R. 2004. Changes in fat and lean body mass during androgen-deprivation therapy for prostatic cancer. *Urology* 63(4):742-725.

Stafford, R. S., and P. L. Cyr. 1997. The impact of cancer on the physical function of the elderly and their utilization of health care. *Cancer* 80(10):1883-1886.

SUPPORT Principal Investigators. 1995. A controlled trial to improve care for seriously ill hospitalized patients. The study to understand prognoses and preferences for outcomes and risks of treatments. *Journal of the American Medical Association* 274(20):1591-1598.

Sweeney, C., K. H. Schmitz, D. Lazovich, B. A. Virnig, R. B. Wallace, and A. R. Folsom. 2006. Functional limitations in elderly female cancer survivors. *Journal of the National Cancer Institute* 98(8):504-505.

Taplin, S. H., W. Barlow, N. Urban, N. T. Mandelson, D. J. Timlin, L. Ichikawa, and P. Nefcy. 1995. Stage, age, comorbidity, and direct costs of colon, prostate, and breast cancer care. *Journal of the National Cancer Institute* 87(6):417-426.

U.S. Census Bureau. 2005. Current Population Reports, P23-209, 65+ in the United States: 2005. Washington, DC: U.S. Government Printing Office.

WHO (World Health Organization) Expert Committee. 1990. *Cancer pain relief and palliative care.* Geneva, Switzerland: WHO Technical Report Series, No. 804.

Yancik, R.1997a. Epidemiology of cancer in the elderly: Current status and projections for the future. *Rays* 22(suppl 1):3-9.

Yancik, R. 1997b. Integration of aging and cancer research in geriatric medicine. *Journals of Gerontology Series A: Biological Sciences and Medical Sciences* 52(6):M329-M332.

Yancik, R., and M. E. Holmes. 2002. *Exploring the role of cancer centers in integrating aging and cancer research.* NIA/NCI Report of Cancer Center Workshop June 13-15, 2001. http://www.nia.nih.gov/ResearchInformation/ConferencesAndMeetings/ WorkshopReport/ExecutiveSummary.htm (accessed December 29, 2006).

Yancik, R., M. N. Wesley, L. A. Ries, R. J. Havlik, B. K. Edwards, and J. W. Yates. 2001. Effect of age and comorbidity in postmenopausal breast cancer patients aged 55 years and older. *Journal of the American Medical Association* 285(7):885-892.

Appendix

Workshop Agenda

Institute of Medicine
National Cancer Policy Forum
The Keck Center of the National Academies
500 5th Street, NW
Keck 201
Washington, D.C. 20001
October 30, 2006

8:00 am   Monday, October 30, 2006, at the Keck Center, Room 201
Continental Breakfast

8:30 am   Welcome, Opening Remarks, and Approval of Minutes
ACS/IOM Breast Cancer and Smoking Workshop—Update
and Approval
Discussion of Forum's 3rd year
Updates—HIPAA, Biomarkers
March Meeting Agenda (Genetic Counseling, Molecular
Imaging, Other?)
Sarcoma Referrals
Harold Moses and staff

9:20 am   Cancer in the Elderly—Introduction
Patricia Ganz and Betty Ferrell

9:30 am   The U.S. Demographic Imperative: Implications for
Oncology Practice
Rosemary Yancik, National Institute of Aging

10:10 am Clinical and Delivery System Issues—Comorbidity and
          Quality of Care
          Rebecca Silliman, Boston University

10:50 am Break

11:00 am Cancer Rehabilitation
          Stephanie Studenski, University of Pittsburgh

11:40 am Nursing Roles and Capacity
          Deborah Boyle, Banner Good Samaritan Medical Center

12:20 pm Lunch

1:15 pm   Family Caregiving
          Barbara Given, Michigan State

1:55 pm   End-of-Life Care
          Kathleen Foley, Memorial Sloan-Kettering

2:35 pm   Economics of Cancer in the Elderly Population
          Tina Shih, MD Anderson Cancer Center

3:15 pm   Research Issues
          *Ann O'Mara, NCI; Rosemary Yancik, NIA representative; Jerry
          Yates, American Cancer Society*

4:00 pm   Concluding Remarks and Adjourn
          Harold Moses